NATURAL WEIGHT LOSS SUPPLEMENT FOR WOMEN:

The Natural Path to Women's Weight Loss and Wellness | Everything You Need to Know About Natural Weight Loss Supplements.

TINA BROOKS

COPYRIGHT

All rights reserved. No part of this publication may be reproduced, distributed, or transmitted in any form or by any means, including photocopying, recording, or other electronic or mechanical methods, without the prior written permission of the publisher, except in the case of brief quotations embodied in critical reviews and certain other noncommercial uses permitted by copyright law.

TABLE OF CONTENTS

INTRODUCTION

As women, the journey to lose weight can be a challenging one due to societal standards and physical changes. However, there is hope with "Natural Weight Loss Supplements for Women." This book offers practical strategies that prioritize well-being and fit into even the busiest schedules. By embracing body diversity, respecting individuality, and following natural rhythms, readers will discover the science behind natural supplements and how to incorporate them into a holistic lifestyle.

Armed with knowledge, resources, and a positive perspective, women can make informed decisions about their health and celebrate every step toward their goals. Achieving a healthy weight can be a challenging journey for women due to societal pressures and physiological changes. "Natural Weight Loss Supplements for Women" offers sustainable weight loss strategies that prioritize well-being and seamlessly integrate into busy lives.

The goal is to empower women with knowledge, tools, and insights to make informed decisions about health and celebrate progress toward achievable milestones.

CHAPTER 1

Understanding Natural Supplements

Natural supplements are items manufactured from natural sources, such as herbs, plants, minerals, and other naturally occurring components. They are generally eaten orally in the form of capsules, pills, powders, or liquids, to give extra nutrients, boost health, and treat particular health conditions. These supplements may comprise vitamins, minerals, amino acids, antioxidants, and botanical extracts.

On the other hand, pharmaceutical items are often synthetic or chemically produced molecules designed for particular medicinal uses. They undergo thorough testing, research, and regulatory approval before being recommended by healthcare experts. Pharmaceutical medications are typically used to treat, manage, or prevent medical disorders, and they may have significant impacts on the body owing to their focused modes of action.

The key distinctions between natural supplements and pharmaceutical medications include:

1. Source and Composition

Natural supplements are obtained from natural sources, whereas pharmaceutical medications are created in labs. Supplements normally comprise a variety of several natural chemicals, whereas medications frequently consist of a single active agent.

2. Regulation

Natural supplements are regulated as dietary supplements, which have fewer strict standards than pharmaceutical medications. This implies that their safety, effectiveness, and quality control may vary. Pharmaceutical medications go through lengthy clinical testing and regulatory procedures before approval.

3. **Intended Use**

Natural supplements are generally used to enhance overall health, cover nutritional shortages, or offer holistic well-being. Pharmaceutical medications are developed to treat particular medical disorders, with defined doses and interactions.

4. **Mechanism of Action**

Natural supplements tend to act more gradually by giving nutrients that may be deficient in the diet. Pharmaceutical medications have well-defined mechanisms of action, targeting particular biochemical pathways to generate desired medicinal effects.

5. **Negative Effects and Interactions**

Natural supplements often have fewer documented negative effects compared to pharmaceutical medications. However, they may still interact with drugs and have possible detrimental effects, especially when taken in high doses.

6. **Prescription**

Natural supplements are frequently accessible over the counter without a prescription. Pharmaceutical medications, on the other hand, need a prescription from a qualified healthcare professional.

It's vital to realize that both natural supplements and pharmaceutical goods have their responsibilities and advantages. While natural supplements are typically used for general well-being and nutritional support, pharmaceutical medications serve a key role in treating medical disorders and illnesses.

Let's look more into the numerous aspects leading to the increased interest in natural methods of health and wellness:

1. **Preventive Treatment**

The growth in chronic illnesses and lifestyle-related health conditions has led to a change in emphasis from reactive to proactive treatment. Natural practices, such as keeping a balanced diet, participating in regular exercise, and managing stress, are gaining popularity as individuals learn that adopting preventative steps may greatly affect their overall health.

2. Minimal Intervention

The need for therapies with fewer side effects and invasiveness has pushed people to investigate natural solutions. Unlike pharmaceutical treatments that could come with possible hazards and difficulties, natural therapies frequently hold a reputation for gentler interventions that function in unison with the body's processes.

3. Holistic Wellness

Modern civilization understands the necessity to handle health as a complex notion. Natural treatments correspond with this holistic vision, realizing that well-being comprises not just physical health but also mental and emotional elements. People are increasingly pursuing methods that create a healthy and fulfilled living.

4. **Personalized Health**

Individuals are learning that health is complicated and distinctive to each individual. Natural techniques allow the freedom to personalize health programs according to one's requirements, tastes, and circumstances. This individualized approach connects with consumers who desire healthcare solutions that correspond with their personalities.

5. **Transparency and Empowerment**

The internet era has allowed people to access a variety of information on health and wellbeing. This has led to a need for openness in healthcare choices, leading consumers to study alternative cures, diet, and lifestyle habits. Empowered with information, people may make educated decisions regarding their well-being.

6. **Cultural and Historical Influence**

Many ancient healing approaches have endured the test of time and are firmly ingrained in many cultures. As individuals strive to connect with their past and accept ancestral knowledge, interest in natural medicines, herbal therapies, and holistic practices has skyrocketed, bridging the gap between old traditions and contemporary well-being.

7. Environmental Awareness

The worldwide push towards sustainability and eco-conscious living has extended to health decisions. Natural techniques generally coincide with ecologically friendly activities, appealing to those who want their health endeavors to be in harmony with the world.

8. Growth of the Wellness Sector

The wellness sector has expanded from a niche market to a mainstream one. The industry today encompasses an assortment of natural goods and services, such as organic foods, herbal supplements, yoga retreats, meditation applications, and wellness-focused vacation experiences. This increase indicates the desire for different and comprehensive well-being alternatives.

9. An Integrative Approach

The merging of natural and conventional methods of treatment is gaining popularity. Recognizing the complementary nature of these treatments, healthcare professionals are partnering across disciplines to provide patients with a full and well-rounded approach to their health.

10. Study and Education

Scientific study has begun to establish the advantages of natural methods to health and wellbeing. As evidence-based information becomes more available, people are better positioned to make educated decisions about adopting natural practices into their lifestyles. This rising corpus of evidence helps debunk myths and increases trustworthiness.

In essence, the increased interest in natural methods of health and wellness implies a paradigm change in the way people see and pursue their well-being. It expresses a common goal for a more proactive, individualized, and holistic approach to health that resonates with both individual needs and larger societal ideals.

Benefits of Using Natural Supplements for Weight Loss

Dietary supplements include chemicals that are swiftly absorbed by the body and alter the internal processes to exhibit benefits.

In the same manner, the top weight reduction products in the market operate in the following three methods.

1. Burn More Calories
Weight loss pills enhance your metabolic rate. During this process, the food you ingest is transformed into energy by burning calories.

2. Suppress Appetite
Weight loss pills reduce your appetite. This helps you feel full after consuming small

amounts of food and makes it simpler for you to remain in a caloric deficit condition.

3. Reduce Fat Absorption

Some supplements lessen the amount of fat and calories absorbed from your dietary intake. This instantly inhibits your body from turning those calories into fat cells.

In summary, weight reduction supplements work by helping you limit your food intake, absorb less fat from it, and burn through your calories quicker.

But that's not all.

Weight loss supplements also provide some important advantages that make them popular.

So, what are these advantages?

Improves your Metabolism

Weight reduction medications and supplements improve the pace at which your body burns calories. This indicates that you have a greater metabolic rate than typical during exercise and other regular activities. This also helps you digest meals more rapidly, burning up even more calories in the process.

You have Greater Energy

With an enhanced metabolic rate comes better energy levels. This helps you remain active and alert throughout the day without feeling fatigued. With a large energy reserve, you don't get fatigued quickly and can work out better and for longer.

Help Control Food Cravings

Weight loss pills function as appetite suppressants. This implies that you eat less and feel full sooner. This is a terrific strategy to make sure your servings are regulated and you don't give in to food cravings. You also maintain this sensation of contentment for a longer duration without feeling hungry.

Stabilized Blood Sugar Levels

Fluctuations in blood sugar levels may lead to cravings and energy dumps, which can impede weight reduction attempts. Some natural substances, like cinnamon and chromium, have been examined for their capacity to help manage blood sugar levels. By encouraging stable blood sugar, these vitamins lead to higher energy levels and fewer cravings.

Inflammation Reduction
Chronic inflammation in the body has been related to weight gain and metabolic abnormalities. Natural supplements high in antioxidants, such as curcumin and omega-3 fatty acids, offer anti-inflammatory qualities that may help minimize this risk. By reducing inflammation, these vitamins encourage a healthy metabolic environment.

Balanced Hormones
Hormonal variations, especially those connected to menstrual cycles and menopause, might affect weight control in women. Some natural supplements, such as maca root and black

cohosh, have been advised to assist balance hormones and reduce symptoms that can impair weight reduction progress.

Keeps you in a Cheerful Mood

When your metabolism is running effectively and your previous meal is keeping you feeling full and content, being in a good mood comes easily. Apart from this, most weight reduction pills also include additional compounds such as antioxidants, vitamins, caffeine, etc. that are known to have mood-boosting advantages.

You Burn Fat even when Resting

Weight loss pills and fat burners try to enhance your resting metabolic rate. Your body continues to burn calories at a greater rate even after you're done exercising. This implies that you burn calories even when you're resting, watching TV, or even taking a nap.

Psychological Well-Being

Successful weight reduction goes beyond physical changes—it's also about psychological well-being. Natural supplements like Rhodiola rosea and ashwagandha have adaptogenic characteristics that may help manage stress and create a happy mentality, minimizing emotional eating triggers.

Note of Caution
While natural supplements provide potential advantages, it's vital to approach them with a balanced attitude. Not all supplements are appropriate for everyone, and individual reactions might vary. Before adopting any new supplement into your regimen, speak with a healthcare practitioner to confirm its compatibility with your health profile.

How can Natural Supplements Aid Metabolism, Appetite Control, and Overall Well-Being

Natural supplements may play a role in improving metabolism, hunger management, and general well-being via several processes. Here's how they may influence each of these aspects:

Boosting Metabolism for Efficient Weight Loss

Metabolism is the cornerstone of energy expenditure and weight regulation. Some natural supplements include bioactive substances that have been related to improved metabolic rates. Green tea extract, for example, includes catechins that may enhance thermogenesis—the process of creating heat and burning calories. This impact might lead to a steady decline in body weight over time.

Curbs Appetite and Reduce Cravings

Controlling appetite and controlling cravings are key components of effective weight reduction. Natural supplements like Garcinia cambogia and 5-HTP alter the release of hormones that control fullness. By generating a sensation of fullness and pleasure, these supplements help lower the chance of overeating and emotional eating, which commonly impair weight reduction attempts.

Promoting Stable Blood Sugar Levels

Blood sugar variations may lead to energy dumps and sugar cravings, limiting weight reduction success. Supplements like cinnamon and chromium have been examined for their ability to control blood sugar levels. By avoiding spikes and crashes, these vitamins help to prolong energy and decrease food cravings.

Balancing Hormones for Optimal Weight Control

Hormonal abnormalities, especially linked to menstruation and menopause, might affect weight control in women. Certain natural supplements, such as maca root and black cohosh, contain adaptogenic characteristics that assist in normalizing hormonal changes. This balance enhances general well-being and may indirectly help weight reduction attempts.

Fostering a Positive Mindset and Stress Management

Psychological well-being is intimately connected to effective weight reduction. Natural supplements having adaptogenic characteristics, such as Rhodiola rosea and ashwagandha, aid in controlling stress and creating a pleasant attitude. By lowering stress-induced cravings and emotional eating triggers, these vitamins help to a healthy relationship with food.

Complementary Role of Natural Supplements

It's crucial to remember that although natural supplements provide these potential advantages, they perform best when incorporated into a holistic strategy for weight management. Their effects are best when accompanied by a balanced diet, frequent physical exercise, and conscious self-care. Moreover, individual reactions to supplements might differ, underlining the need for individualized methods to attain the greatest outcomes.

Scientific Basis of Natural Supplements

The efficacy of natural supplements isn't anchored in anecdotal experiences alone. Robust scientific study gives insights into how particular bioactive substances inside supplements interact with the body's metabolic processes. Studies done on animals, cells, and people add to our knowledge of the processes via which these supplements exert their benefits.

Green Tea Extract and Metabolism

Green tea extract, rich in catechins including epigallocatechin gallate (EGCG), has received interest for its ability to enhance metabolism. Research shows that EGCG may boost thermogenesis by increasing energy expenditure and fat oxidation. Studies have indicated moderate gains in weight reduction when green tea extract is integrated into a balanced weight management plan.

Garcinia Cambogia and Appetite Management

Garcinia cambogia, which contains hydroxycitric acid (HCA), has been examined for its impact on appetite management. Some studies show that HCA may suppress an enzyme involved in turning excess carbs into fat. While data are inconsistent, several studies have indicated moderate decreases in body weight and hunger in persons taking Garcinia cambogia pills.

Cinnamon and Blood Sugar Management

Cinnamon, recognized for its unique taste, has shown potential in improving blood sugar management. Compounds like cinnamaldehyde and procyanidins in cinnamon may promote insulin sensitivity and glucose utilization.

Although findings vary, research shows that integrating cinnamon into the diet might lead to better blood sugar control.

Maca Root and Hormonal Balance

Maca root, an adaptogenic plant, has been related to hormonal balance and well-being. While studies are continuing, some evidence shows that maca may impact hormone levels and lessen symptoms connected to hormonal swings. By improving balance, maca root might indirectly improve weight control attempts caused by hormonal shifts.

Evidence-Informed Decisions

It's crucial to view scientific research with a critical eye. Studies may differ in design, sample size, and length, resulting in conflicting conclusions. Moreover, individual reactions to supplements might vary depending on variables including heredity and lifestyle. Consulting reliable sources, such as peer-reviewed publications and expert reviews, may help you make evidence-informed judgments.

Holistic Integration

As we investigate the scientific foundation of natural supplements, remember that they are most successful when incorporated into a holistic approach to well-being. While research gives insights, the complexity of human physiology demands a multimodal approach that combines supplements with balanced eating, frequent physical exercise, and conscious self-care.

In the chapters ahead, we will continue to dig into particular natural supplements, analyzing their possible advantages, effects, doses, and concerns. By integrating scientific insights with practical help, we seek to empower you to make educated decisions that correspond with your health objectives.

Importance of Evidence-Based Information

The capacity to discern between true efficacy and mere conjecture is vital, particularly when it comes to natural supplements. This section looks into the relevance of relying on evidence-based information when contemplating the inclusion of supplements into your weight reduction journey.

Navigating the Sea of Claims

The area of natural supplements is replete with bold declarations and promises of miraculous effects. Yet, not everything that glitters is gold. Relying on evidence-based information serves as a compass to navigate through the sea of claims, helping you to make educated decisions anchored in study and science.

Foundation of Credibility

Evidence-based information is established in rigorous scientific research. Studies are aimed at studying the effects of supplements on the human body via controlled experimentation, observation, and data analysis. Such research creates the cornerstone of credibility, offering insights into the processes, benefits, and possible hazards linked with particular supplements.

Discerning Fact from Fiction

By finding evidence-based knowledge, you empower yourself to distinguish fact from fiction. Peer-reviewed scientific publications, expert reviews, and clinical trials are trustworthy sources that give impartial assessments of supplement effectiveness. These sources undergo extensive inspection by specialists in the subject, confirming the credibility of the information they give.

Understanding Mechanisms of Action

Evidence-based research goes beyond surface-level claims and digs into the underlying mechanisms of action that underpin supplement benefits. Understanding how a supplement interacts with the body's metabolic processes helps you to appreciate its possible advantages and limits. This information helps you to make decisions that match your health objectives.

Mitigating Health Concerns

Supplements, like any intervention, contain the potential for both benefits and concerns. Evidence-based information supplies you with the skills to analyze the safety of supplements. For example, knowing about possible interactions with drugs or health problems helps you make educated choices that preserve your well-being.

Consulting Healthcare Professionals

The relevance of evidence-based knowledge becomes more obvious when considering your health profile. Consultation with healthcare specialists, such as physicians, certified dietitians, or nutritionists, ensures that supplement selections are suited to your unique requirements. They can help you comprehend scientific results and propose supplements that match your overall health strategy.

Holistic Approach to Wellbeing

Integrating supplements into your weight loss journey is most beneficial when done within the framework of a holistic approach to wellbeing. Evidence-based information acts as a guidepost, aiding you in choosing decisions that complement a balanced diet, frequent physical exercise, and mindfulness practices.

By accepting evidence-based information, you empower yourself with the knowledge required to make decisions that connect with your well-being and objectives.

The Importance of Consulting with Healthcare Professionals

Embarking on a path to include natural supplements in your weight reduction program is an empowering move. However, this route is best followed with the aid of healthcare specialists. Let's discuss the necessity of getting professional counsel before incorporating supplements into your regimen.

Personalized Guidance for Your Health Profile

No two persons are alike in their health requirements, concerns, or medical history. When you speak with a healthcare expert, such as a doctor or registered dietitian, you're able to analyze your health profile holistically. They assess issues such as pre-existing illnesses, allergies, prescriptions, and possible combinations. This guarantees that the vitamins you purchase are suited to your well-being.

Mitigating Risks and Adverse Effects

Supplements, especially those taken from natural sources, may entail risks and possible adverse effects. Healthcare providers are qualified to inform you about possible hazards, contraindications, and interactions. Armed with this information, you're able to make educated decisions that limit the chance of bad impacts.

Navigating Complex Interactions

Many folks use prescription drugs, which might interact with supplements. Healthcare experts possess a detailed grasp of these interactions and can advise you in picking supplements that are compatible with your prescriptions. This advice avoids unforeseen outcomes that might harm your health.

Monitoring Progress and Adjustments

A fundamental benefit of working with healthcare experts is their ability to assess your progress over time. Regular check-ins enable them to examine how supplements are influencing your health and alter recommendations appropriately. This dynamic method guarantees that your supplement regimen changes with your changing demands.

Balancing Holistic Wellness

Healthcare experts evaluate your health through a holistic lens, taking into consideration physical, mental, and emotional well-being. Their advice goes beyond supplement selection—it involves balanced eating, physical exercise, stress management, and general well-being. This holistic viewpoint guarantees that your health journey is thorough and sustainable.

Empowered by Information for Informed Choices

By receiving help from healthcare experts, you arm yourself with information that empowers your decision-making. You acquire a greater grasp of the possible advantages and limits of supplements within the context of your entire health plan. This educated approach creates confidence and responsibility in your fitness journey.

The relationship between you and your healthcare provider is a partnership in your well-being. Their knowledge matches your aims, resulting in well-informed decisions that connect with your goals.

Interactions with Drugs and Health Problems

It's crucial to realize that supplements, although frequently helpful, have the potential to interact with drugs and health problems. This section sheds light on the necessity of knowing these interactions before taking supplements in your weight reduction quest.

The Complexity of Biochemical Interactions

Our bodies are complicated biochemical systems where diverse chemicals interact. Natural supplements provide unique substances that may impact how drugs are digested and used. These encounters might be pleasant, bad, or even neutral, underscoring the need for care and awareness.

Medication-Supplement Interactions

Certain supplements may interact with prescription or over-the-counter drugs. For instance, St. John's wort, commonly taken for mood support, might diminish the efficiency of various antidepressants. Supplements like omega-3 fatty acids could alter blood-thinning drugs. These encounters underline the significance of contacting healthcare specialists to minimize unforeseen outcomes.

Health Condition Considerations

Individuals with certain health issues need to take more care while using supplements. For instance, those with renal difficulties should be careful of supplement amounts that can strain kidney function. Similarly, those with bleeding issues need to be careful with substances that alter blood coagulation.

Consult Healthcare Professionals

By explaining your health profile and prescription regimen, you allow them to discover possible interactions and propose supplements that correspond with your overall health plan.

Transparent Communication

When consulting healthcare experts, transparent communication is crucial. Provide complete information about the drugs you're taking, including dose and frequency. Disclose any underlying health conditions or sensitivities. This information allows healthcare experts to deliver individualized recommendations that emphasize your well-being.

Balancing the Advantages

While interactions are a factor, it's crucial to find a balance between the possible advantages of supplements and the necessity to prevent dangers. Healthcare experts can help you make educated decisions that optimize the advantages of supplements while limiting the chance of interactions that might endanger your health.

Supplementing Responsibly

Interactions between supplements and medications/health problems underline the significance of a careful and educated approach to supplementing. By contacting healthcare specialists, you ensure that your supplement selections correspond with your overall health objectives without weakening current therapies or health issues.

A joint Approach

The inclusion of supplements into your weight reduction journey should be considered as a joint initiative between you and healthcare providers. Their knowledge ensures that you manage possible encounters with care and confidence, helping you to make decisions that promote your well-being.

Regulation and Quality Control Across Regions

The worldwide landscape of natural supplements is distinguished by variances in legislation and quality control requirements across various areas. Let's investigate the unique measures adopted by various nations to guarantee the safety, effectiveness, and quality of supplements.

Varied Regulatory Frameworks

Regulation of natural supplements varies greatly from one nation to another. Some areas have strong rules that categorize supplements as a sort of medicine, requiring extensive testing and approval. In contrast, some nations classify supplements as nutritional goods, resulting in varied degrees of control.

United States: Dietary Supplement Health and Education Act (DSHEA): In the United States, the DSHEA defines dietary supplements and puts out laws controlling their labeling, safety, and claims. While producers are responsible for assuring product safety, the FDA intervenes only once safety problems develop. This regulatory approach lays a degree of duty on customers to make educated decisions.

European Union: Novel Food Regulations: The European Union utilizes the Novel Food Regulation, which controls novel and innovative food items, including supplements. Before a new supplement can be brought to the market, it undergoes a comprehensive study to establish its safety. This method stresses pre-market review to avoid possible dangers.

Canada: Natural Health Products Regulations: Canada's Natural Health Products Regulations concentrate on pre-market evaluation and post-market monitoring. These requirements require producers to present proof of safety, effectiveness, and quality before a supplement may be marketed. Post-market monitoring tries to detect and resolve safety risks that can occur after a product is on the market.

Australia: Therapeutic Products Administration (TGA): Australia's TGA regulates therapeutic products, including supplements. The TGA analyzes safety, quality, and effectiveness before goods are put on the market. Manufacturers must present proof to back their claims, ensuring that supplements fit with recognized criteria.

Quality Control and Good Manufacturing Practices (GMP): Regardless of regional variances in legislation, quality control and adherence to Good Manufacturing Practices (GMP) are necessary. GMP guidelines provide methods for production, testing, and quality assurance. Brands that comply with GMP standards exhibit a dedication to creating safe and effective supplements.

Informed Consumer Choice: Understanding the regulatory landscape of supplements in your location empowers you as a customer. Be aware of legislation controlling product claims, labeling, and safety. Rely on respected companies that value quality control and openness in their production processes.

Navigating other Markets: If you're contemplating supplements from other markets, be aware of the regulatory situation in those locations. Differences in rules may affect product availability, quality, and safety. Research the rules regulating supplements in that nation to make educated judgments.

By being aware of these distinctions, you may make decisions that match your health objectives while emphasizing safety and effectiveness.

Selecting Reputable and High-Quality Supplements

In a market crowded with supplements, discriminating between high-quality selections and substandard goods may be tough. Let's examine helpful advice to assist you through the selection process and pick supplements that are reliable, safe, and effective.

1. Research the Brand

Begin by investigating the brand providing the supplement. Companies that value openness, offer information about their production procedures and have a history of excellent goods are desirable. Ensure they conform to Good Manufacturing Practices (GMP) and undergo third-party testing for purity and potency.

2. Read Labels and Claims

Thoroughly study the supplement's label. Steer careful of items with ambiguous claims or promises that seem too good to be true. Opt for supplements that include clear component lists, correct dosing information, and claims validated by scientific research.

3. Seek Third-Party Testing

Third-party testing gives credibility. Choose supplements that have passed testing by independent labs for quality, purity, and efficacy. Certifications from organizations like NSF International, USP, or ConsumerLab.com demonstrate adherence to strict quality standards.

4. Check for Scientific Backing

Prioritize supplements with scientific research backing. Look for items that reference clinical studies, peer-reviewed publications, or expert evaluations. Scientific confirmation provides legitimacy to a supplement's efficacy and possible advantages.

5. Consult Healthcare Experts

Consult healthcare experts before adopting a new supplement. Doctors, licensed dietitians, or nutritionists may give individualized recommendations based on your health profile and objectives. They aid you in picking supplements that are suitable and safe.

6. Consider Dosage and Form

Exercise cautiously with supplements advertising excessive dosages or extraordinarily high concentrations of active components. Verify whether the dose fits with established standards and if the supplement is available in a form that aids optimum absorption.

7. Evaluate Customer Evaluations

While not the primary factor, customer evaluations might give information. Look for trends in reviews, paying attention to input concerning side effects, advantages, and changes reported by people.

8. Avoid Proprietary mixes

Be wary of supplements stating "proprietary blends." These mixes sometimes don't identify constituent quantities, making it tough to determine effectiveness and safety.

9. Price and Value

Quality supplements may have a premium price, but be aware of unduly inflated costs. Strike a balance between quality and value, evaluating credible solutions that emphasize your health investment.

10. Listen to Your Body

Observe your body's reaction while taking a supplement. If you notice unpleasant effects or unexpected changes, see your healthcare provider and consider quitting the supplement.

Being an educated consumer and following these suggestions, you select decisions that correspond with your health objectives while prioritizing safety, efficacy, and long-term well-being.

Individual Variability in Response

It's vital to note and remember that individual reactions to supplements might vary greatly depending on various variables, including genetics, lifestyle, and current health issues. Here's why individualized results are an important consideration when utilizing natural supplements:

1. Genetic Variability

Our genetic composition determines how our bodies absorb and react to different things, including supplements. Genetic variances may affect how well a supplement is absorbed, digested, and used by the body. As a consequence, what works well for one individual may not have the same impact on another.

2. Metabolic Diversity

Metabolism differs from individual to person. Factors including age, gender, and metabolic rate might impact how fast or slowly the body reacts to supplements. Some people could see immediate effects, while others may take more time to detect any changes.

3. **Existing Health Disorders**

Underlying health disorders may dramatically affect how the body reacts to supplements. Certain health problems may increase or lessen the effects of supplements, and in certain situations, supplements might even mix with drugs, leading to undesired results.

4. **Diet and Lifestyle**

A person's diet and lifestyle choices have a key impact on how supplements are absorbed and used. A well-balanced diet rich in nutrients might boost the efficiency of supplements, while bad dietary habits could hamper their effects. Similarly, frequent exercise and good lifestyle choices might lead to improved results.

5. **Biochemical Individuality**

Each person has a distinct biochemical constitution, resulting in variances in food demands and reactions. What works ideally for one person's body chemistry could not correspond with another's, resulting in varied outcomes from the same substance.

6. **Placebo Effect**

Psychological variables might impact perceived supplement efficacy. The placebo effect, when a person perceives favorable changes owing to the belief in a treatment's effectiveness, might alter outcomes. Personal views and expectations may impact how someone experiences the effects of a supplement.

7. **Amount and length**

The amount and length of supplement administration might also affect results. Some supplements may take constant usage over a lengthy time to exhibit obvious results, while others could offer fast improvements at lesser dosages.

8. **Interactions and Tolerance**

The interaction between supplements and other substances, including drugs, herbs, and meals, might impact how they perform in the body.

Additionally, an individual's tolerance to various supplements might vary, leading to diverse experiences and consequences.

Determining Appropriate Dosages for Different Supplements

Understanding how to calculate suitable quantities for various supplements is vital to guarantee you're receiving the advantages without jeopardizing your health. Let's discuss techniques to aid you in choosing the proper dose for your requirements.

1. Refer to Scientific Research

Scientific research frequently gives insights into optimal doses for certain supplements. Look for research-backed suggestions in credible publications and expert evaluations. Keep in mind that doses might vary depending on the supplement's intended function and the target group of the research.

2. **Start with Recommended Doses**

Many supplements come with recommended doses on the package. These doses are typically based on research and are deemed safe for the average person. Starting with the prescribed dose might give a great basis for examining how your body reacts.

3. **Consider Your Goals**

The goal of taking a supplement determines the optimal dose. For example, if you're taking a supplement for general well-being, you could follow a different dose than if you're using it for particular health objectives like weight reduction or immune support. Align the dose with your goals.

4. **Account for Individual Factors**

Factors like age, gender, weight, heredity, and current health issues have a part in choosing the proper dose for you. Individual variability implies that what works for one person cannot work the same way for another. Consulting healthcare specialists helps customize doses to your requirements.

5. Look for Dosage Ranges

In certain circumstances, supplements contain a range of effective dosages rather than a single suggested dosage. This variety reflects the variance in individual reactions. Start at the lower end of the range and progressively raise as required, under expert advice.

6. Adjust Based on Response

Listen to your body's instincts while taking supplements. If you get favorable benefits at the prescribed dose, you may not need to raise it. Conversely, if you're not getting the intended outcomes or are having ill effects, try reducing the dose or quitting the supplement.

7. Consult Healthcare Experts

The experience of healthcare experts is crucial for choosing proper doses. Doctors, licensed dietitians, and nutritionists may examine your health profile and objectives to propose doses matched to your requirements. Their counsel avoids needless dangers.

8. Be Wary of Excessive Doses

While supplements might bring advantages, excessive doses can lead to unwanted consequences. More is not always better. Stick to specified doses and resist the urge to overdo them in the expectation of quicker results. Remember that moderation is crucial.

9. Monitor Over Time

Even after finding an acceptable dose, continue monitoring your body's reaction. Factors such as changes in lifestyle, health state, or objectives could demand dose modifications. Regular check-ins with healthcare specialists assist in ensuring your dose stays acceptable.

10. Prioritize Safety and Efficacy

When choosing suitable doses, prioritize safety and efficacy. Striking the appropriate mix between the two guarantees you're maximizing the advantages of supplements while preserving your health.

Following Prescribed Dosage Recommendations

When it comes to adding supplements into your health routine, according to prescribed dosage recommendations is crucial. This section digs into the relevance of following these rules to guarantee safety, efficacy, and best outcomes.

Safety First

Recommended use recommendations are established with safety in mind. By following recommendations, you limit the danger of negative results and emphasize your well-being.

Avoiding Unnecessary Risks

More isn't always better when it comes to supplements. Deviating from established use recommendations raises the probability of developing adverse effects or surpassing safe levels. Abiding by these principles helps you avoid avoidable dangers that might harm your health.

Optimizing Effectiveness

Supplements are created with appropriate doses to achieve desired effects. Following prescribed use standards guarantees that you're supplying your body with vital nutrients in the proper quantities. This optimization boosts the chance of attaining your specified health objectives.

Preventing Diminished Returns

Taking large doses of supplements does not always correlate to improved outcomes. It may lead to decreasing returns or even nullify the intended advantages. By following suggested doses, you preserve the balance essential for supplements to perform properly.

Avoiding Interactions

Supplements, like pharmaceuticals, may interact with one another or with current health concerns. Following prescribed use recommendations helps avoid interactions that might adversely influence your health. This careful approach is especially necessary if you're taking many vitamins or drugs concurrently.

Professional Approval

Healthcare experts typically make dose recommendations based on your health profile. Disregarding their recommendations and exceeding suggested doses might weaken their knowledge and the tailored approach they give to assist your well-being.

Maintaining Long-run Sustainability

Supplement regimens should be sustainable over the long run. Abiding by prescribed use recommendations guarantees that you're ingesting supplements in a way that supports your body's ongoing health demands without producing strain or imbalances.

Listening to Your Body

Even while following rules, it's crucial to listen to your body's indications. If you notice unexpected symptoms or changes, see healthcare providers and consider modifying your regimen. Your body's response helps fine-tune your strategy for the best outcomes.

Balancing Patience and Progress

Patience is a virtue when it comes to supplements. Consistently following prescribed use recommendations enables you to notice development over time without hurrying or expecting fast benefits. This balanced approach accords with the notion of comprehensive well-being.

Key Takeaways

In this chapter, we've looked into the diverse world of natural supplements and their potential to help your weight reduction journey. Let's highlight the major lessons that underline the necessity of making educated and responsible decisions when incorporating supplements into your health regimen:

1. Research and Reputable Companies

Prioritize companies that are honest about their production procedures, adhere to Good production procedures (GMP), and undergo third-party testing for quality and purity. A recognized brand is the cornerstone of your supplement adventure.

2. Guided by Science

Choose supplements that are backed by scientific research and confirmed by clinical trials, peer-reviewed publications, or expert evaluations. Scientific data provides credibility to a supplement's efficacy and advantages.

3. Consult Healthcare Specialists

Before introducing new supplements, consult with healthcare specialists. Their experience offers individualized recommendations based on your health profile, ensuring your decisions correspond with your overall well-being.

4. Right Doses

Determine the right doses for various supplements by referring to scientific research, beginning with suggested dosages, and evaluating your health objectives and specific variables. Balance is crucial to enhancing performance.

5. Follow Usage Rules

Adhering to approved usage rules is vital. Doing so assures safety, minimizes needless risks, maximizes efficacy, and prevents interactions with other vitamins or prescriptions.

6. Individual Responses Differ

Understand that individual responses to supplements might differ depending on genetics, lifestyle, and underlying health concerns. Embrace an adaptive strategy that incorporates your physiology.

7. Patience and Progress

Supplements are not a shortcut but a tool to support your health journey. Balancing patience with development enables you to achieve durable outcomes and avoid possible problems.

8. Holistic Well-Being

Approach supplements as part of a holistic wellness strategy that includes balanced eating, regular physical exercise, stress management, and general well-being. Supplements are one part of your holistic health approach.

9. Empowerment Through Information

Empower yourself with information to make educated judgments. By incorporating supplements deliberately, led by specialists, and in sync with your body's response, you go on a path of better health and energy.

10. Responsibility and Well-Being

Ultimately, the educated and responsible use of natural supplements adds to your well-being. By navigating the supplement environment with insight and care, you take command of your health path with confidence and purpose.

The decisions you make today have the ability to influence a healthier and more vibrant future.

CHAPTER 2

Key Natural Supplements for Weight Loss

As we go into particular natural supplements recognized for their help in the domain of weight reduction, it's crucial to grasp the distinct contributions each supplement makes. These supplements, supported by scientific study, have garnered a reputation for their ability to assist your weight control journey. Let's analyze how each supplement plays a part in promoting weight reduction while highlighting the necessity of appropriate supplementing.

Green Tea Extract

Green tea extract has emerged as a popular alternative in the search for weight reduction. Its high amount of catechins, notably epigallocatechin gallate (EGCG), provides it with metabolic-boosting and fat oxidation capabilities. Catechins induce thermogenesis, improving calorie expenditure even during rest. Additionally, green tea extract's capacity to alter hormones involved in hunger and fullness provides appetite control advantages. Research shows that including green tea extract in your routine may encourage a more efficient metabolism and enable better eating behaviors, leading to lasting weight reduction.

Garcinia Cambogia

Garcinia cambogia contains hydroxycitric acid (HCA) and has received interest for its ability to decrease fat accumulation and lower hunger. HCA's action includes inhibiting an enzyme that assists in turning excess carbs into fat, perhaps diverting them for energy consumption. This impact, along with appetite-suppressing qualities, makes Garcinia Cambogia a competitor in weight control regimens. However, it's vital to approach its utilization with care, considering individual reactions and possible interactions.

Conjugated Linoleic Acid (CLA)

Conjugated linoleic acid (CLA) is a fatty acid present in meat and dairy products. It has earned notoriety for its function in retaining lean muscle mass while boosting fat reduction. CLA seems to impact enzymes involved in fat accumulation and breakdown, leading to healthier body composition. Research shows that CLA may promote fat reduction, especially in resistant places like the belly, by boosting metabolism and changing body composition. Integrating CLA into your routine may complement exercise efforts and aid in sustained weight control.

Forskolin

Forskolin, produced from the Coleus forskohlii plant, has shown promise in aiding weight reduction via its impact on cyclic adenosine monophosphate (cAMP) levels. Increased cAMP levels drive cellular mechanisms that boost fat breakdown and metabolic rate. Forskolin's capacity to boost the body's sensitivity to hormonal cues may lead to more successful weight reduction attempts. However, like with any supplement, knowing the dose and individual differences is vital for getting the desired benefits.

Raspberry Ketones

Raspberry ketones, chemicals responsible for the scent of raspberries, have gained interest for their possible influence on adiponectin, a hormone involved in metabolism and fat breakdown. While research is continuing, several studies show that raspberry ketones may boost fat oxidation and lower hunger. These effects position raspberry ketones as possible friends in assisting weight reduction initiatives.

Yet, intelligent supplementation, along with a complete approach to health, remains vital.

Caffeine

Caffeine, a well-known stimulant found in coffee and tea, may also have a role in weight reduction. Its effects on energy expenditure, fat oxidation, and appetite control have made it a popular element in weight loss pills. Caffeine activates the neurological system, boosting metabolism and accelerating the breakdown of accumulated lipids. Its influence on alertness may also boost physical performance, adding to calorie expenditure during exercise. However, moderation is vital, recognizing individual tolerances and avoiding excessive use.

Apple Cider Vinegar

Apple cider vinegar has garnered attention for its ability to affect weight control via its acetic acid concentration. Acetic acid may alter metabolism, lowering fat accumulation, and blood sugar increases after meals. Incorporating apple cider vinegar into your routine may give appetite management advantages and aid in more steady energy levels throughout the day. As with any supplement, prudent use and expert assistance are crucial for maximizing its potential advantages.

Glucomannan

Glucomannan, produced from the konjac root, is a soluble fiber noted for its extraordinary capacity to absorb water and induce a sense of fullness. By expanding in the stomach, glucomannan may control appetite and decrease calorie intake. Its effect in inducing fullness and lowering overeating makes it a helpful tool in weight control efforts. Ensuring optimal dose and timing is key for enhancing glucomannan's efficacy.

Emphasizing Evidence-Based Choices

The value of evidence-based decision-making cannot be emphasized. When contemplating natural supplements for weight reduction, depending on trustworthy scientific data becomes your compass, directing you toward options that correspond with your health objectives. Here's why evidence-based knowledge should be your guiding light:

1. **Differentiating Fact from Fiction**
The supplement business may be filled with marketing promises that seem intriguing but lack scientific support. Evidence-based information helps you sort through the noise, helping you to discern between assertions established in robust studies and those that are simple suppositions.

2. **Validating usefulness**
Scientific studies give a prism through which you may analyze a supplement's usefulness. Peer-reviewed research gives insights into how a

supplement interacts with the body, its methods of action, and its potential advantages. This validation supplies you with the information required to make educated decisions.

3. **Gauging Safety and Risks**
Evidence-based information not only throws light on prospective advantages but also tackles safety issues. Scientific studies may reveal possible hazards, interactions with other drugs, and unwanted consequences. This information helps you to make decisions that emphasize your well-being.

4. **Personalization and Individual Variability**
Human physiology differs from person to person. Evidence-based research takes into consideration individual reactions to supplements, letting you understand if a supplement is likely to work for you based on scientific evidence rather than generic promises.

5. **A full view**

Evidence-based information gives a full view of a supplement's effect. It analyzes long-term impacts, possible interactions, and the larger context of health and well-being. This comprehensive vision helps you to make decisions consistent with your total well-being.

6. Informed Conversations with Experts

When equipped with evidence-based information, you may participate in meaningful conversations with healthcare experts. Sharing your supplement selections and the scientific basis behind them enables specialists to give individualized counsel that takes into account your specific health profile.

7. Long-Term Sustainability

Weight control is not a short-term undertaking but a lifetime commitment to health. Evidence-based decisions encourage sustainable practices that endure the test of time. By picking supplements based on sound research, you establish a basis for your health journey.

8. **Confidence in Your Choices**

Choosing evidence-based supplements instills confidence in your judgments. You're not just following trends; you're making decisions informed by knowledge and motivated by the desire for actual health improvement.

Let's dive into the details of the aforementioned natural supplements now, shall we?

Green Tea Extract

Benefits of Green Tea Extract for Weight Loss: Metabolism-Boosting Marvel

Green tea extract has emerged as a star performer in the arena of weight control, garnering attention for its varied variety of possible advantages. One of its most appreciated features resides in its metabolism-boosting abilities, which contribute greatly to its function in promoting weight reduction.

1. **Metabolism Amplification**

Green tea extract owes its metabolism-boosting abilities to its substantial amount of catechins, notably epigallocatechin gallate (EGCG). Catechins are bioactive chemicals that exhibit strong effects on cellular processes, increasing metabolism and encouraging calorie expenditure even at rest. The metabolic rate is the energy your body expends to sustain fundamental operations including breathing, digesting, and circulation. By boosting this rate, green tea extract efficiently promotes the energy-burning process.

2. **Enhanced Fat Oxidation**

EGCG, the major catechin in green tea extract, has been found to improve fat oxidation, or the breakdown of stored fat for energy. This process includes the conversion of stored triglycerides into free fatty acids that may be used by cells. Green tea extract increases this conversion, allowing the usage of fat reserves for energy generation, which is important in weight reduction attempts.

3. **Thermogenesis Stimulation**

Thermogenesis refers to the development of heat inside the body. It's a process that happens when your body consumes calories to create energy and maintain temperature. Green tea extract's catechins, mainly EGCG, have been implicated with increasing thermogenesis. This impact leads to an increase in calorie expenditure, as the body expends greater energy to create heat. By boosting thermogenesis, green tea extract aids weight reduction by contributing to greater energy expenditure.

4. **Fat reduction from Stubborn Parts**

Certain parts of the body, frequently referred to as "stubborn fat areas," tend to store fat more quickly and might be tough to target with traditional weight reduction approaches. Green tea extract has demonstrated promise in assisting fat reduction from certain places, such as the abdominal region. By stimulating metabolism and accelerating fat breakdown, green tea extract may help people attain more balanced fat distribution and healthier body composition.

5. Satiety Support

Another feature of green tea extract's significance in weight control resides in its capacity to impact hunger regulation. Catechins, notably EGCG, have been examined for their influence on hormones implicated in appetite and satiety, such as ghrelin and leptin. While research is continuing, several studies show that green tea extract may help manage appetite and minimize overeating, leading to a lower calorie intake.

Potential Side Effects of Green Tea Extract: Considerations for Safe Usage

While green tea extract provides several advantages for weight control, it's crucial to note that like any supplement, it may come with possible adverse effects. Being aware of these possible negative effects allows you to make responsible decisions and prioritize your well-being.

1. Caffeine Sensitivity

Green tea extract includes caffeine, but at lesser levels compared to a cup of brewed coffee. Individuals sensitive to caffeine may have symptoms such as jitteriness, anxiety, elevated heart rate, or sleep difficulties. If you are very sensitive to caffeine, it's suggested to monitor your reaction and explore low-caffeine or caffeine-free options.

2. Gastrointestinal Distress

In certain situations, green tea extract may cause gastrointestinal discomfort, including stomachache, nausea, or diarrhea. These effects may vary from person to person and may be impacted by variables like dose and individual tolerance. Starting with a smaller dosage and gradually increasing it may help decrease the chance of severe pain.

3. Interactions with drugs

Green tea extract has the potential to interact with certain drugs. It may alter the absorption or efficacy of pharmaceuticals such as blood thinners, antidepressants, and some cardiac medications. If you are using prescription drugs, contact a healthcare practitioner before introducing green tea extract into your routine to ensure safety and avoid any interactions.

4. Liver Health Concerns

In rare circumstances, excessive use of green tea extract has been connected with liver-related issues. While these situations are unusual, it's essential to take care, particularly if you have pre-existing liver issues or if you're taking drugs that impair liver function. Regular monitoring and visiting a healthcare expert are advised.

5. Iron Absorption

Green tea extract includes substances known as tannins that may hinder the absorption of non-heme iron, the kind of iron found in plant-based meals. If you have low iron levels or depend on plant-based sources of iron, be careful of this possible interaction. Consider spacing out ingestion of green tea extract from iron-rich meals to improve iron absorption.

Green tea extract's metabolism-boosting characteristics position it as a helpful weapon in your weight control armory. By increasing metabolism, improving fat oxidation, and stimulating thermogenesis, green tea extract promotes your body's natural mechanisms that lead to weight reduction.

It's also vital to approach supplements with mindfulness and awareness. Potential side effects are not universal, and many people have no harmful effects. However, acknowledging the possible hazards and being alert to your body's reaction ensures that you go on this adventure with a balanced viewpoint.

Guidance on Dosages and Proper Usage of Green Tea Extract

As you continue on your path to harness the potential advantages of green tea extract for weight control, knowing the optimum quantities and proper administration is vital to assure both safety and efficacy. Here's a guide to assist you in navigating the area of green tea extract supplementation:

1. Start Low and Gradually Increase

When adding any new supplement to your regimen, including green tea extract, it's wise to start with a smaller amount. This strategy enables your body to adjust and decreases the danger of any negative effects. Begin with a dosage of roughly 250 to 500 mg of green tea extract each day.

2. Consider Caffeine Content

Green tea extract naturally includes caffeine, but at lesser levels compared to a cup of coffee. If you are sensitive to caffeine or use other sources of caffeine during the day, consider this when deciding your green tea extract dose. Opting for decaffeinated versions or spacing out intake may be useful.

3. Pay Attention to Standardization

Look for green tea extract supplements that contain standardized quantities of catechins, notably epigallocatechin gallate (EGCG). Standardization guarantees that you're obtaining consistent and predictable amounts of the active components that contribute to its potential advantages.

4. Timing Matters

Consider taking your green tea extract supplement with meals to prevent any stomach discomfort. Dividing your regular dosage into numerous smaller doses throughout the day may also assist in boosting absorption and lessen the probability of gastrointestinal irritation.

5. Expert Guidance

Consulting a healthcare expert before introducing green tea extract into your routine is encouraged, particularly if you have current health concerns or are using prescription drugs. A healthcare practitioner may make individualized suggestions based on your health profile and guarantee that there are no possible interactions.

6. Monitor Your Response

As you begin consuming green tea extract, pay attention to how your body reacts. Note any changes in energy levels, appetite, and general well-being. Monitoring your reaction helps you assess if the dose is suitable and whether any changes are required.

7. Stay Hydrated

Green tea extract may have a slight diuretic effect, perhaps leading to increased urine production. Staying well-hydrated throughout the day is vital to maintain optimal hydration levels.

8. **Complement with a Balanced Lifestyle**
While green tea extract may play a part in weight control, it's vital to note that supplements are most successful when incorporated into a comprehensive strategy. Prioritize a balanced diet, frequent physical exercise, and appropriate sleep to maximize your weight control journey.

Finding the proper dose that corresponds with your body's reaction and objectives demands time and awareness. By emphasizing expert assistance, addressing individual sensitivities, and promoting a total wellness approach, you prepare the path for the best outcomes.

Garcinia Cambogia

Garcinia cambogia, a tropical fruit native to Southeast Asia, has received interest for its possible advantages in weight control. Central to its attractiveness are its qualities that impact both appetite reduction and the inhibition of fat storage—a combination that places Garcinia cambogia as a fascinating ally in the search for successful weight loss.

Appetite Suppression Mechanism

At the core of Garcinia Cambogia weight management potential lies hydroxycitric acid (HCA), a natural chemical found in the fruit's rind. HCA is considered to alter appetite control via multiple mechanisms:

1. Serotonin modification

HCA has been connected with the modification of serotonin levels in the brain. Serotonin is a neurotransmitter that plays a major function in mood and appetite control. By possibly boosting serotonin levels, HCA may lead to an enhanced feeling of well-being and a decrease in emotional eating.

2. Regulation of Ghrelin Levels

Garcinia cambogia may also alter the levels of ghrelin, widely referred to as the "hunger hormone." Ghrelin informs the brain when it's time to eat, and greater levels are related to increased hunger. Some studies show that HCA may help manage ghrelin levels, leading to decreased appetite and a reduced desire to overeat.

3. Inhibition of Fat accumulation

Beyond its effects on hunger, Garcinia cambogia is considered to have a function in reducing fat accumulation. This is primarily related to HCA's interaction with an enzyme called citrate lyase:

4. Citrate Lyase Inhibition

Citrate lyase is an enzyme involved in the conversion of excess carbs into fat. HCA is considered to decrease the action of citrate lyase, possibly shifting carbs toward energy generation instead of fat storage. By limiting this enzyme's function, Garcinia cambogia may aid in the prevention of new fat buildup.

5. Shift in Energy Utilization

When citrate lyase activity is inhibited, the body is urged to utilize carbs for immediate energy demands rather than turning them into fat. This adjustment in energy use may promote a more effective metabolism and lead to a lower probability of excess fat accumulation.

Potential Side Effects of Garcinia Cambogia Supplementation: Considerations for Safe Usage

While Garcinia cambogia has attracted attention for its possible weight management advantages, it's crucial to realize that like any product, it may come with potential negative effects. Being aware of these possible adverse effects helps you to make educated choices and prioritize your well-being.

1. Gastrointestinal Discomfort

Some persons may suffer gastrointestinal discomfort, including stomachache, bloating, or diarrhea, after using Garcinia cambogia pills. These effects may vary from person to person and may be impacted by variables like dose and individual tolerance. Starting with a smaller dosage and gradually increasing it may help decrease the chance of severe pain.

2. Interactions with Certain Drugs

Garcinia cambogia supplements have the potential to interfere with certain drugs, particularly those used for diabetes management and cholesterol control. The supplement may impact blood sugar levels and lipid profiles, demanding care if you're using medicine for these illnesses. Consult with a healthcare practitioner before introducing Garcinia cambogia into your diet, particularly if you're on prescription drugs.

3. Potential Liver Concerns

In rare situations, Garcinia cambogia consumption has been connected with liver-related issues. While occurrences of these consequences are unusual, it's advised to take care, especially if you have pre-existing liver issues or if you're taking drugs that impair liver function. Regular monitoring and expert supervision are needed.

4. Allergic Reactions

Individuals with sensitivities to Garcinia cambogia or other members of the Clusiaceae family should exercise care while contemplating supplementation. Allergic reactions, however rare, may include skin rashes, itching, or breathing problems. If you have known allergies, speak with a healthcare practitioner before taking Garcinia cambogia pills.

5. Impact on Pregnancy and Nursing

Limited information is known on the safety of Garcinia cambogia supplementation during pregnancy and nursing. Due to the possible hazards and ambiguities, pregnant and nursing persons are recommended to avoid Garcinia cambogia supplements and seek assistance from a healthcare expert.

6. Expert assistance and individualized Considerations

The possible adverse effects of Garcinia cambogia underline the significance of expert assistance and individualized considerations. Before integrating this supplement into your routine, particularly if you have underlying health concerns or are using drugs, check with a healthcare provider. They may give insights into possible interactions, assist you in evaluating the appropriateness of supplementing, and direct you toward responsible decisions.

Individual reactions might vary considerably. While many people have no detrimental effects, prudent use and educated judgments are crucial.

Dosing Recommendations and Considerations for Safe and Effective Use of Garcinia Cambogia

The world of supplements demands a balanced strategy that balances safety, effectiveness, and individual concerns in order to avoid issues.

Here are some suggestions and key aspects to keep in mind:

1. **Recommended Dosage Range**

The recommended dosage of Garcinia cambogia extract might vary depending on the number of active components, notably hydroxycitric acid (HCA). In general, doses generally fall within the range of 500 to 1500 mg of Garcinia cambogia extract per day, with HCA concentrations ranging from 50% to 60%. However, it's crucial to follow the particular dose guidelines specified on the supplement package.

2. **Gradual Introduction**

When commencing Garcinia cambogia supplementation, it's best to begin with a lesser dose and gradually increase it. This strategy enables your body to acclimatize and decreases the danger of any negative effects. Starting with the lower end of the suggested dose range is a wise option.

3. **Expert Guidance**

Consulting a healthcare expert before introducing Garcinia cambogia into your routine is highly encouraged, particularly if you have pre-existing health concerns, are using medicines, or are pregnant or nursing. A healthcare expert may examine your particular health profile and make individualized advice suited to your requirements.

4. **Monitor Your Response**

As you introduce Garcinia cambogia, pay attention to how your body reacts. Note any changes in appetite, energy levels, and general well-being. Monitoring your reaction helps you assess if the recommended dose is beneficial for you and whether any changes are required.

5. **Avoid Excessive intake**

Excessive intake of Garcinia cambogia pills does not always lead to greater outcomes and may raise the risk of negative effects. Stick to the stated doses and avoid exceeding them without expert assistance.

6. Cycling and Breaks

To minimize any tolerance or habituation, try cycling your Garcinia cambogia intake. This comprises periods of supplement usage followed by pauses. Consulting with a healthcare expert may help you develop a suitable cycling routine.

7. Comprehensive Approach

Remember that supplements are most effective when incorporated into a comprehensive approach to well-being. Prioritize a balanced diet, frequent physical exercise, hydration, and proper sleep with Garcinia cambogia supplements for total weight control.

8. Quality Matters

Choose high-quality Garcinia cambogia products from reputed producers. Look for products that have standardized HCA content and comply with quality and purity requirements.

Conjugated Linoleic Acid (CLA)

A Dual-Action Ally for Body Fat Reduction and Muscle Preservation

Conjugated Linoleic Acid (CLA) is a kind of fatty acid that has attracted interest for its possible influence on body composition. Widely found in meat and dairy products from grass-fed animals, CLA is famous for its dual-action effects in lowering body fat while retaining lean muscle mass—a combination that makes it an attractive candidate in the domain of weight control.

Body Fat Reduction Mechanisms

CLA's capacity to promote body fat reduction is hypothesized to be anchored in various mechanisms:

1. **Lipogenesis Inhibition**
CLA may limit lipogenesis, the process by which the body turns excess dietary

carbohydrates into fat for storage. By blocking this process, CLA possibly lowers the formation of new fat and maintains a caloric balance that favors weight reduction.

2. Lipolysis Stimulation

Lipolysis, the breakdown of stored triglycerides into free fatty acids for energy usage, is a significant component of fat loss. CLA is considered to induce lipolysis, improving the mobilization of stored fat to be utilized as fuel.

3. Modulation of Fat-Burning Enzymes

CLA is considered to affect enzymes involved in fat metabolism, such as carnitine palmitoyltransferase (CPT). By modulating these enzymes, CLA may promote the use of fatty acids for energy generation, adding to total fat reduction.

Preservation of Lean Muscle Mass

What sets CLA distinctive is its ability to help in maintaining lean muscle mass along the weight reduction journey:

1. Metabolic Impact

Lean muscle mass is metabolically active tissue that contributes to calorie expenditure even at rest. CLA's impact on body composition entails prioritizing the consumption of fat for energy while preserving lean muscular tissue. This metabolic advantage helps avoid the loss of lean muscle that might occur with fast weight reduction.

2. Impact on Protein Synthesis

CLA may also boost protein synthesis—a process necessary for maintaining and growing muscular tissue. By increasing protein synthesis, CLA ensures that the body retains the essential resources to protect muscular integrity.

3. Potential Hormonal Influence

CLA's effects on hormones, such as growth hormone and insulin sensitivity, are considered to have a role in sustaining lean muscle mass. These hormonal interactions lead to an environment favorable to preserving muscle while losing fat.

By leveraging CLA's dual-action advantages, you pave the path for a balanced change that coincides with your health and well-being ambitions.

Potential Side Effects of Conjugated Linoleic Acid (CLA) Supplementation: Understanding the Considerations

While Conjugated Linoleic Acid (CLA) has promise as a natural supplement for weight control, it's vital to be aware of any negative effects that may result from its consumption. As you ponder adopting CLA into your health journey, here are some key points to bear in mind:

1. **Stomach Distress**

Some persons may develop stomach pain after using CLA supplements. This pain might show as stomachache, bloating, gas, or diarrhea. Starting with a lower dosage and gradually increasing it may help lessen the chance of gastrointestinal side effects.

2. Potential Insulin Resistance

In rare situations, CLA supplementation has been linked with a slight loss in insulin sensitivity. While the influence seems to be mild and varies across people, those with diabetes or insulin-related issues should exercise caution and contact a healthcare expert before contemplating CLA supplementation.

3. Impact on Blood Lipids

Research has indicated that CLA supplementation may alter blood lipid profiles, including changes in cholesterol levels. While the effects are typically minor, those with established cardiovascular issues should obtain advice from a healthcare specialist before taking CLA supplements.

4. **Potential Allergic responses**

As with any supplement, there is a chance of allergic responses to CLA. Individuals with documented sensitivities to safflower oil or other similar substances should approach CLA supplementation carefully. If you have any allergy symptoms, such as skin rash or breathing difficulties, cease usage and see a healthcare expert.

5. **Interactions with drugs**

CLA supplements may interact with some drugs, including anticoagulants (blood thinners), diabetic medications, and immunosuppressants. If you are on any prescription drugs, speak with a healthcare provider before considering CLA supplementation to verify there are no possible interactions.

6. **Potential Impact on Liver Function**

In rare situations, CLA supplementation has been connected with deleterious effects on liver function. If you have existing liver issues or are on drugs that influence liver function, see a healthcare provider before using CLA supplements.

7. Hormonal Influence

CLA's influence on hormones, notably estrogen levels, is a field of current study and inquiry. If you have hormone-related illnesses or concerns, talk with a healthcare physician before contemplating CLA supplementation.

Dosing Strategies and Potential Interactions:

Knowing proper dose techniques and possible interactions with other supplements is crucial to ensure a safe and productive experience. Let's discuss dosage concerns and interactions that might impact your CLA supplement experience:

1. Dosing Strategies

Start Gradually: Begin with a lesser dose of CLA and gradually raise it over time. This strategy enables your body to acclimatize and decreases the danger of any negative effects. Most CLA supplements contain dosages ranging from 1000 to 3000 mg per day, split into many doses.

Monitor Response: Pay careful attention to how your body reacts to CLA supplementation. Note any changes in appetite, energy levels, and general well-being. Adjust the dose as required, depending on your body's reaction.

speak practitioner Guidance: Before commencing CLA supplementation, speak with a healthcare practitioner. They may examine your specific health profile, propose the right dose, and give direction on how CLA fits into your entire wellness strategy.

2. Interactions with Other Supplements

Omega-3 Fatty Acids: CLA and omega-3 fatty acids both belong to the family of polyunsaturated fatty acids. While they have unique advantages, their interaction may alter how they are digested. Consult with a healthcare physician if you're contemplating supplementing with both CLA and omega-3 fatty acids.

Fat-Soluble Vitamins: CLA supplements are commonly taken alongside dietary fats to increase absorption. However, excessive ingestion of fat-soluble vitamins (A, D, E, K) plus CLA may raise the risk of vitamin poisoning. Balance your fat-soluble vitamin intake and try spacing out their ingestion.

Diabetic drugs: CLA's possible influence on insulin sensitivity may interact with diabetic drugs. If you're using drugs for diabetic treatment, talk with a healthcare physician before introducing CLA into your routine.

Antiplatelet drugs: CLA's impact on blood clotting mechanisms may interfere with antiplatelet drugs. Consult with a healthcare physician if you're taking antiplatelet medicines such as aspirin or clopidogrel.

L-Carnitine: Both CLA and L-carnitine are related to fat metabolism. While they have separate mechanisms, consider discussing the concurrent use of CLA and L-carnitine with a healthcare professional.

Comprehensive Approach: CLA is most effective when incorporated into a comprehensive approach to well-being. Prioritize a balanced diet, frequent physical exercise, hydration, and proper sleep with CLA supplementation for overall weight control.

By adopting a calibrated dosage plan, monitoring your body's reaction, and being aware of possible interactions, you develop a framework for maximizing the advantages of CLA while reducing dangers.

Forskolin

Forskolin, produced from the roots of the Indian coleus plant (Coleus forskohlii), has emerged as a natural supplement with the potential to impact metabolism and help fat reduction. The compound's unique modes of action have caught the interest of researchers and people seeking effective and comprehensive ways to weight control.

1. Activation of Adenylate Cyclase

One of forskolin's signature mechanisms resides in its ability to activate an enzyme called adenylate cyclase. This activation causes a cascade of processes inside cells that result in higher levels of cyclic adenosine monophosphate (cAMP). Elevated cAMP levels serve a critical role in boosting many physiological responses, including metabolic enhancement and fat breakdown.

2. Enhanced Metabolic Rate

Forskolin's influence on cAMP levels results in heightened metabolic activity. A higher metabolic rate expends more calories even at rest, adding to greater calorie expenditure throughout the day. This metabolic surge is especially useful in the context of weight control since it stimulates the utilization of stored energy reserves—namely, fat.

3. Lipolysis Stimulation

Forskolin's impact extends to the activation of hormone-sensitive lipase—a crucial enzyme responsible for beginning lipolysis, the breakdown of stored triglycerides into free fatty acids. By increasing lipolysis, forskolin increases the escape of fatty acids from adipose tissue, making them accessible for energy consumption.

4. Thermogenesis Promotion

Thermogenesis—the generation of heat inside the body—plays a vital role in calorie expenditure. Forskolin's influence on cAMP levels has been connected to the enhancement of thermogenesis, thereby improving calorie burning. This thermogenic action adds to the total energy deficit necessary for fat reduction.

5. Lean Body Mass Preservation

In addition to encouraging fat reduction, forskolin's capacity to retain lean body mass sets it distinct. While weight loss attempts generally lead to a decrease in both fat and muscle, forskolin's processes appear to prefer the preservation of lean muscle tissue. This preservation is critical for maintaining a healthy metabolism and avoiding metabolic slowing.

6. Appetite Regulation

Emerging evidence shows that forskolin may potentially alter hunger management via interactions with hormones like leptin and ghrelin. By altering hunger hormones, forskolin leads to a more balanced ratio between caloric intake and expenditure.

Possible Side Effects of Forskolin Supplementation

While forskolin has promise as a natural supplement for weight control, it's crucial to be aware of any negative effects that may result from its consumption. As you investigate the possible advantages of forskolin, it's vital to understand the factors for a safe and educated experience:

1. Gastrointestinal Distress
Some people may develop gastrointestinal pain while using forskolin pills. This pain might show as stomach distress, nausea, or diarrhea. Starting with a lower dose and gradually increasing it may help lessen the chance of gastrointestinal side effects.

2. Potential Blood Pressure Effects

Forskolin's effect on cellular pathways may potentially alter blood pressure. While some research shows that forskolin may promote healthy blood pressure levels, others have reported modest decreases or variations in blood pressure. If you have current blood pressure issues, visit a healthcare physician before contemplating forskolin supplementation.

3. Potential Heart Rate Changes

Forskolin's impact on cellular processes may potentially extend to heart rate regulation. Individuals who are sensitive to changes in heart rate or those with pre-existing cardiac issues should exercise care and seek expert counsel before taking forskolin supplements.

4. Potential Interaction with Drugs

Forskolin supplements may interfere with drugs that impact blood pressure, heart rate, and blood coagulation. If you're on antihypertensive meds, antiplatelet pharmaceuticals, or blood thinners, check with a healthcare provider before introducing forskolin into your routine.

5. **Alter on Hormones**

Forskolin's influence on cAMP levels may potentially alter hormonal pathways. While this is crucial to its potential advantages, it's vital to approach supplementing with prudence, especially if you have hormone-related problems or concerns.

6. **Allergic Responses**

As with every product, there is a chance of allergic responses to forskolin. Individuals with documented sensitivities to Coleus forskohlii or other similar substances should approach forskolin administration carefully. If you encounter any allergy reactions, cease usage and see a healthcare expert.

7. **Practitioner Guidance**

Given the possible interactions and individual variances, consultation with a healthcare practitioner before contemplating forskolin supplementation is highly suggested. A healthcare practitioner may examine your health profile, identify possible hazards, and give individualized counsel based on your particular requirements.

While possible side effects exist, it's vital to understand that individual reactions might vary greatly.

Optimizing Dosages and Usage Patterns

Achieving the best outcomes with forskolin supplements needs a deliberate approach to dosing and use patterns. As you continue on your path to harness the potential advantages of forskolin, consider the following advice to optimize its influence on your weight control efforts:

1. Consult Professional Assistance

Before commencing forskolin supplementation, obtain assistance from a healthcare practitioner. A healthcare practitioner may examine your health profile, consider any current diseases or drugs, and propose a suitable dose customized to your unique requirements.

2. Start Conservatively

Begin with a smaller dose of forskolin to examine your body's reaction. This careful approach enables you to measure your tolerance and limit the danger of any negative effects. A normal initial dose may vary from 25 to 50 mg per day.

3. Gradually Increase Dose

If your body reacts well and you have no unwanted effects, try gradually increasing the dose over time. A usual dosage range for forskolin supplementation is between 50 and 250 milligrams per day, split into two to three doses.

4. Monitor Response

Pay special attention to how your body responds to forskolin supplementation. Note changes in energy levels, appetite, and general well-being. Monitoring your reaction helps you to make educated choices about altering doses and use habits.

5. Cyclic Usage Patterns

Consider adopting cyclic usage patterns while utilizing forskolin. For example, you may utilize forskolin for several weeks, followed by a time of cessation. This method helps prevent the body from acquiring resistance to the supplement's effects.

6. Combination with Lifestyle Factors

Forskolin's potential advantages are amplified when incorporated with a healthy lifestyle. Prioritize a good diet, frequent physical exercise, water, and appropriate sleep. Forskolin complements these elements and adds to a comprehensive approach to weight control.

7. Hydration and Timing

Stay hydrated when taking forskolin, since optimal hydration helps metabolic processes. Take forskolin pills with meals to increase absorption and limit the risk of unwanted gastrointestinal discomfort.

8. Professional Monitoring

Regularly interact with your healthcare physician while utilizing forskolin. They may review your progress, monitor any changes in health indicators, and give recommendations on altering doses if required.

By speaking with a healthcare practitioner, beginning slowly, monitoring your reaction, and incorporating forskolin into a holistic wellness strategy, you build a foundation for optimizing the potential advantages of this natural supplement.

Raspberry Ketones

Their Impact on Fat Metabolism and Weight Reduction

Raspberry ketones, the aromatic chemicals responsible for the characteristic scent of raspberries, have received interest for their possible function in promoting fat metabolism and weight loss. These substances are considered to impact different physiological processes that contribute to a comprehensive approach to weight control.

1. Enhancement of Lipolysis

Raspberry ketones are considered to enhance lipolysis—the breakdown of stored triglycerides into free fatty acids. By promoting lipolysis, raspberry ketones contribute to the release of fatty acids from adipose tissue, making them accessible for energy consumption. This procedure corresponds with the greater objective of increasing fat reduction.

2. Release of Adiponectin

Adiponectin, a hormone generated by adipose tissue, plays a vital function in regulating glucose metabolism and fatty acid oxidation.

Raspberry ketones are suspected to alter adiponectin levels, perhaps enhancing its release. Higher levels of adiponectin are related to greater insulin sensitivity and enhanced fat metabolism.

3. Increased Fat Oxidation

The influence of raspberry ketones on adiponectin secretion is accompanied by an increase in fat oxidation. Fat oxidation includes the conversion of fatty acids into energy via biological mechanisms. By boosting fat oxidation, raspberry ketones lead to increased calorie expenditure, producing an environment beneficial to weight loss.

4. Potential Appetite Regulation

Emerging evidence shows that raspberry ketones may alter hunger management via interactions with hormones like leptin. Leptin is a hormone that conveys feelings of fullness and modulates food intake. By altering leptin sensitivity, raspberry ketones may have a role in reducing cravings and fostering mindful eating.

5. Preservation of Lean Body Mass

One of the remarkable properties of raspberry ketones is their ability to enhance the retention of lean body mass during weight reduction. While the primary aim is fat loss, retaining lean muscle tissue is vital for a healthy metabolism and general well-being.

How Raspberry Ketones Influence Fat Cells

The effects of raspberry ketones on fat cells are assumed to be a consequence of complicated chemical interactions that influence many physiological processes. As we look into the probable methods by which raspberry ketones impact fat cells, a clearer picture develops of their function in aiding weight control.

Enhancement of Hormone Sensitivity

Raspberry ketones are considered to boost the sensitivity of fat cells to hormones that govern metabolism and fat breakdown. One such hormone is adiponectin, which plays a vital role in insulin sensitivity and fatty acid oxidation. By boosting adiponectin levels and strengthening its signaling, raspberry ketones lead to a more effective fat metabolism.

Stimulation of Lipolysis

Lipolysis, the process by which stored triglycerides are broken down into free fatty acids, is a vital step in fat reduction. Raspberry ketones are considered to induce lipolysis inside fat cells. This stimulation leads to the release of fatty acids from adipose tissue, making them accessible for energy consumption.

Activation of Hormone-Sensitive Lipase

Raspberry ketones may also stimulate an enzyme called hormone-sensitive lipase (HSL), which is important to starting lipolysis. HSL's activation kicks off a chain reaction that dismantles triglycerides into free fatty acids. The released fatty acids may subsequently be transferred to other cells for energy synthesis.

Increase in Adiponectin Secretion

Adiponectin, generated by fat cells, has a function in regulating insulin sensitivity and metabolic balance. Raspberry ketones are considered to stimulate the release of adiponectin from fat cells. This hormone promotes fat breakdown and utilization while also generating an anti-inflammatory environment.

Influence on Gene Expression

Raspberry ketones can impact the expression of genes associated with metabolism and fat oxidation. This effect occurs at the genetic level, altering the development of enzymes and proteins involved in energy expenditure and fat utilization.

Thermogenesis Stimulation

Raspberry ketones are also known to boost thermogenesis—a process in which the body creates heat and expends energy. By activating genes involved in thermogenesis, raspberry ketones lead to greater calorie burning, further assisting in weight control efforts.

Potential Side Effects of Raspberry Ketones Supplementation

While raspberry ketones offer promise as a natural supplement for weight control, it's crucial to be aware of any adverse effects that may result from its consumption. As you explore adding raspberry ketones into your health program, here's a complete look at the factors for a safe and educated experience:

1. Gastrointestinal Discomfort

Some persons may suffer gastrointestinal discomfort, such as stomach upset, nausea, or diarrhea, after using raspberry ketones tablets.

Starting with a lower dose and gradually increasing it may help lessen the chance of gastrointestinal side effects.

2. Potential Allergic Response

As with any supplement, there is a chance of allergic responses to raspberry ketones. Individuals with documented sensitivities to raspberries or similar substances should approach raspberry ketone supplementation carefully. If you encounter any allergy reactions, cease usage and see a healthcare expert.

3. Interaction with Caffeine

Raspberry ketones may interact with caffeine, perhaps enhancing the effects of caffeine. If you consume a substantial quantity of caffeine from other sources, consider adjusting your caffeine consumption while utilizing raspberry ketones.

4. Blood Pressure and Heart Rate Effects

Given the possible impact on metabolism and hormonal interactions, raspberry ketones may have effects on blood pressure and heart rate. If you have pre-existing blood pressure problems or cardiac disorders, see a healthcare practitioner before integrating raspberry ketones into your diet.

5. Practitioner Assistance

Before commencing raspberry ketones supplementation, obtain assistance from a healthcare practitioner. A healthcare practitioner may examine your health profile, consider possible combinations with drugs or current diseases, and give individualized advice on use.

6. Hormonal Considerations

Raspberry ketones' effect on hormonal pathways may affect persons with hormone-related illnesses. If you have hormonal abnormalities or concerns, consider the possible advantages and hazards of raspberry ketones with a healthcare specialist.

7. Monitoring and Self-Awareness

As you utilize raspberry ketones supplements, keep a high sense of self-awareness. Monitor how your body reacts, notice any changes in energy levels, appetite, and general well-being, and be prepared to reduce doses or quit treatment if required.

While possible side effects exist, it's crucial to realize that individual reactions might vary greatly.

Dosages and Usage for Raspberry Ketones

Knowing doses and use patterns is vital for a safe and productive experience. Here's a thorough resource to help you explore the world of raspberry ketones:

1. Start with Professional Guidance

Before commencing raspberry ketones supplementation, see a healthcare professional. They may examine your health profile, consider any current diseases or drugs, and propose a suitable dose customized to your unique requirements.

2. **Begin Conservatively**

Commence your raspberry ketones adventure with a cautious approach. Start with a smaller dose to observe how your body reacts. A normal initial dose may vary from 100 to 200 mg per day.

3. **Gradual Increase**

If your body reacts well and you encounter no unwanted effects, try gradually increasing the dose over time. A usual range for raspberry ketone supplementation is between 200 and 600 mg per day, split into two or three dosages.

4. **Monitor and Adjust**

Monitor your body's reaction attentively as you raise the dose. Note any changes in energy levels, appetite, and general well-being. Adjust the dose as required depending on your body's reaction.

5. **Cyclic Usage Patterns**

To prevent the body from acquiring resistance to raspberry ketones, try adopting cyclic usage patterns. This entails consuming raspberry ketones for many weeks, followed by a period of withdrawal. Consult your healthcare physician for information on the length of use cycles.

6. Synergistic Lifestyle Factors

Raspberry ketones are most effective when incorporated into a comprehensive health strategy. Prioritize a balanced diet, frequent physical exercise, water, and excellent sleep. Raspberry ketones complement these elements and add to a complete weight control plan.

7. Timing and Absorption

Take raspberry ketone supplements with meals to increase absorption and limit the risk of unwanted gastrointestinal discomfort. Staying hydrated is also vital to assist metabolic activities.

8. Professional Oversight

Regularly interact with your healthcare physician while utilizing raspberry ketones. They may monitor your progress, examine any changes in health indicators, and give recommendations on modifying doses if required.

Caffeine

Caffeine, a natural stimulant present in coffee, tea, and other supplements, may promote weight reduction via its effects on energy expenditure and appetite control. Here's how caffeine helps to these two crucial features of weight management:

1. **Energy Expenditure (Thermogenesis):** Caffeine has been demonstrated to have thermogenic qualities, which means it may temporarily raise the body's heat production and metabolic rate. This leads to an enhanced energy expenditure, as the body expends more calories to create heat. The thermogenic properties of

caffeine may help in weight reduction in the following ways:

- Increased Basal Metabolic Rate (BMR): Caffeine may boost the body's resting metabolic rate, which accounts for a large amount of daily calorie expenditure. A higher BMR indicates that the body burns more calories even while at rest.

- Enhanced Fat Oxidation: Research shows that caffeine may promote the breakdown of stored lipids (lipolysis) and the subsequent oxidation of fatty acids for energy. This implies that the body is more prone to utilize fat as a fuel source, especially during activity.

- Physical Performance: Caffeine has been demonstrated to boost exercise performance by improving endurance, strength, and power output. When paired with physical activity, caffeine's performance-enhancing properties may contribute to increased calorie expenditure during workouts.

2. **Appetite Suppression:** Caffeine may also impact appetite control, which is an essential element of weight management. It may alter appetite via numerous mechanisms:

- Central Nervous System Stimulation: Caffeine stimulates the central nervous system, resulting in enhanced alertness and reduced sensations of weariness. This may indirectly alter appetite by lowering the impression of hunger.

- Neuropeptide Regulation: Caffeine intake has been connected with the modification of neuropeptides that control hunger. It may influence hormones including ghrelin (the hunger hormone) and leptin (the satiety hormone), perhaps resulting in decreased sensations of hunger.

- Catecholamine Release: Caffeine increases the release of neurotransmitters including adrenaline (epinephrine) and noradrenaline (norepinephrine). These neurotransmitters may decrease hunger and boost the body's usage of stored energy, including fat.

- Short-Term Suppression: Some persons experience a short-term appetite suppression effect quickly after drinking caffeine. This might lead to lower calorie consumption during meals.

It's crucial to remember that although caffeine might give potential advantages for weight reduction, individual reactions can differ. Additionally, tolerance to caffeine might build over time, thereby decreasing its benefits on energy expenditure and appetite control. Let's delve into the possible side effects.

Exploring Potential Side Effects of Caffeine Consumption

While caffeine may provide several advantages in aiding weight control, it's vital to be aware of possible adverse effects that may emerge from its usage. As you explore introducing coffee into your health regimen, here's an investigation of the possible concerns to bear in mind:

1. Insomnia and Sleep Disturbances

One of the most prevalent negative effects of caffeine usage is impairment in sleep. Caffeine's stimulatory effects might lead to problems falling asleep, staying asleep, or having restorative sleep. To reduce this risk, avoid caffeine use close to sleep.

2. Jitters and Restlessness

Higher doses of coffee may contribute to symptoms of jitteriness, restlessness, and elevated heart rate. If you encounter these symptoms after ingesting coffee, try lowering your dose to a level that your body tolerates easily.

3. Digestive Discomfort

Caffeine may irritate the gastrointestinal system in certain persons, leading to symptoms such as stomach upset, acid reflux, or nausea. Starting with a lesser dose and taking caffeine with meals might help lessen the probability of stomach discomfort.

4. **Increased Heart Rate and Blood Pressure**

Caffeine's influence on the central nervous system might result in higher heart rate and blood pressure. While this is frequently a transitory effect, those with pre-existing cardiac issues or high blood pressure should exercise caution and contact a healthcare practitioner before taking caffeine supplements.

5. **Anxiety and Nervousness**

Sensitive people may feel heightened anxiety, nervousness, or a sensation of uneasiness after taking coffee. If you are prone to anxiety or have a history of anxiety problems, consider monitoring your reaction and modifying your dose appropriately.

6. **Dependence and Withdrawal**

Regular use of caffeine may develop tolerance when the body needs greater dosages to produce the same effects. Abruptly quitting caffeine intake after chronic usage might result in withdrawal symptoms such as headaches, exhaustion, and irritability.

7. Interaction with Drugs

Caffeine may interact with some drugs, possibly decreasing their effectiveness or producing undesired side effects. If you are using drugs, check with a healthcare practitioner before using caffeine supplements to evaluate possible interactions.

8. Individual Variability

It's crucial to note that individual reactions to caffeine may vary substantially. Genetics, tolerance levels, and general health have a crucial effect on how your body responds to caffeine. Monitoring your body's reaction and regulating your usage appropriately is crucial.

As with any dietary modification or supplement, moderation is crucial. If you're contemplating taking caffeine as part of your weight reduction approach, it's essential to see a healthcare practitioner, particularly if you have existing health concerns or are sensitive to caffeine's effects. If you're already hoodwinked into excess consumption of caffeine, every break you get at the office or school, or at night to just be up all night for one thing or the other, it's better you cut down on it. Better safe than sorry.

Combining caffeine consumption with a balanced diet and regular exercise is the most effective and lasting method to reach weight reduction objectives.

Navigating Caffeine Dosing: Personalizing Your Approach for Optimal Results

Effective caffeine administration entails a precise balance between harnessing its advantages and respecting individual tolerance levels. Here's a thorough approach to assist you in understanding optimum dosing:

1. **Start with a Baseline**

When adding coffee into your routine, begin with a baseline dose that fits with your sensitivity to caffeine. A conventional beginning point may be approximately 100 milligrams per day, which is roughly similar to a cup of coffee.

2. Examine Your Response

After drinking caffeine, attentively examine how your body reacts. Note changes in energy levels, alertness, heart rate, and any indications of jitteriness or restlessness. This self-awareness will influence your decision-making when you alter your dose.

3. Gradual Increases

If you discover that your first dose is well-tolerated and you wish greater results, try gradually increasing the dosage over time. Incremental modifications, such as adding 50 milligrams each day, enable you to measure your body's reaction and prevent excessive stimulation.

4. Personal Tolerance Variability

Individual tolerance to caffeine might vary greatly. Factors such as heredity, age, body weight, metabolism, and general health play a part in deciding how your body responds to coffee. What works well for one individual may not be appropriate for another.

5. Avoiding Excessive Use

While caffeine might bring advantages, it's vital to avoid excessive use. Overdosing on caffeine may lead to undesirable consequences such as sleeplessness, anxiety, elevated heart rate, and stomach discomfort. Moderation is crucial.

6. Monitoring Daily Consumption

Be conscious of your entire daily caffeine consumption, including sources outside supplements. Coffee, tea, energy drinks, and even some meals contain caffeine. Keeping track of your cumulative intake helps avoid overconsumption.

7. Adjust Based on Activity Levels

Consider altering your caffeine intake based on your daily activity. If you have a sedentary day, a lesser dose could be sufficient. On days when you participate in greater physical activity, a slightly larger dose can be beneficial.

8. Listen to Your Body
Ultimately, your body's reaction should lead to your caffeine dose selections. If you have unfavorable side effects or discomfort, try lowering your dose or ceasing usage. Prioritize your well-being above anything else.

Navigating caffeine dose is about finding your particular sweet spot—one that gives the required advantages without sacrificing your well-being.

Apple Cider Vinegar

Apple cider vinegar, a fermented liquid generated from apples, has gained recognition for its possible role in assisting weight control.

Let's look into the intriguing ways in which apple cider vinegar may aid in weight reduction and appetite regulation:

1. Appetite Suppression

Apple cider vinegar's impact on appetite management starts with its propensity to induce a sensation of fullness. Acetic acid, a component of apple cider vinegar, has been proven to slow stomach emptying. This implies that food remains in the stomach longer, resulting in a prolonged sense of fullness and decreased appetite.

2. Blood Sugar Balance

Maintaining stable blood sugar levels is vital for weight control. Apple cider vinegar may aid in this area by boosting insulin sensitivity. Improved insulin sensitivity promotes better glucose utilization and reduces spikes and falls in blood sugar levels, which may lead to decreased cravings and improved appetite control.

3. **Improved Digestion**

A healthy digestive system plays a key part in weight control. Apple cider vinegar's acetic acid component may improve digestion by boosting the formation of stomach acid and aiding the breakdown of nutrients. Efficient digestion improves the absorption of nutrients that contribute to overall well-being.

4. **Metabolism Boost**

Apple cider vinegar's possible influence on metabolism resides in its capacity to activate genes that govern fat metabolism. This activation may lead to enhanced fat oxidation and utilization of energy. A heightened metabolism helps with the overall calorie-burning process.

5. **Altered Fat Storage**

Certain animal research shows that apple cider vinegar could impact gene expression associated with fat storage. This shift in gene expression may lead to a decrease in the formation of body fat, especially around the abdominal region.

6. **Reduction In Appetites**

Apple cider vinegar's capacity to regulate blood sugar levels may translate to reduced appetites for sweet and high-calorie meals. By reducing the craving for certain items, people may make more conscious dietary choices that match their weight control objectives.

7. **Supporting Gut Health**

The gut microbiome's role in weight control is widely understood. Apple cider vinegar's prebiotic properties—providing sustenance for healthy gut bacteria—may help to a balanced gut microbiota. A healthy gut ecosystem fosters overall health and well-being.

The potential advantages of apple cider vinegar in weight reduction and appetite management show the extraordinary ways in which natural substances may enhance a holistic approach to well-being.

Acetic Acid's Influence on Metabolism and Blood Sugar Regulation

The acetic acid contained in apple cider vinegar has a vital function in altering metabolism and controlling blood sugar levels. As we look into the numerous ways in which acetic acid affects these physiological systems, a greater understanding develops of its potential advantages in weight management:

1. Blood Sugar Control

Acetic acid's influence on blood sugar control is a characteristic of its potential advantages. When eaten with meals, acetic acid has been found to exhibit a unique impact on post-meal blood sugar levels. It's claimed that acetic acid may slow down the digestion of carbohydrates, resulting in a gradual release of glucose into the circulation. This minimizes fast rises in blood sugar levels and helps maintain more constant glycemic responses.

2. Improved Insulin Sensitivity

Insulin sensitivity, the body's capacity to react to the hormone insulin, is a significant element in blood sugar regulation. Acetic acid has been related to improved insulin sensitivity, which indicates that cells become more sensitive to insulin's actions. This enhanced sensitivity promotes effective glucose absorption by cells, preventing excess glucose from accumulating in the circulation.

3. Enhanced Glucose Consumption

Acetic acid's presence may enhance the effective consumption of glucose by cells for energy generation. By boosting glucose absorption into cells, acetic acid aids in decreasing the total load of glucose circulating in the circulation. This not only promotes blood sugar homeostasis but also lowers the probability of excess glucose being stored as fat.

4. Impact on Fat Metabolism

Acetic acid's impacts on metabolism extend beyond blood sugar management. Research reveals that acetic acid may impact the expression of genes involved in fat metabolism. This influence may lead to enhanced fat oxidation—the breakdown of stored fat for energy consumption. A heightened fat oxidation mechanism adds to total calorie expenditure and improves weight control efforts.

5. Enhanced Satiety

Acetic acid's tendency to prolong gastric emptying—the pace at which food exits the stomach—contributes to heightened sensations of fullness and satiety. This delayed stomach emptying may lead to lower food intake and more regulated eating patterns, further supporting weight management objectives.

The impact of acetic acid in apple cider vinegar on metabolism and blood sugar levels emphasizes its potential as a natural supplement for weight control.

Potential Side Effects: Ensuring a Safe Experience with Apple Cider Vinegar

While apple cider vinegar provides possible advantages for weight control, it's necessary to be aware of any adverse effects that may emerge from its usage. As you contemplate including apple cider vinegar into your health regimen, here's a complete explanation of the possible hazards to bear in mind:

1. Stomach Pain

Apple cider vinegar's acidic nature may cause stomach pain in certain persons. Symptoms such as stomach distress, acid reflux, and heartburn might develop, especially after eating undiluted vinegar. To avoid this danger, it's advised to dilute apple cider vinegar with water before ingestion.

2. Tooth Enamel Erosion

The acidity of apple cider vinegar may also damage dental health. Consuming undiluted vinegar might damage tooth enamel over time. To safeguard your oral health, try using a straw to sip diluted apple cider vinegar and rinse your mouth with water afterward.

3. Blood Sugar Fluctuations

While apple cider vinegar may help manage blood sugar levels, persons who are currently treating diabetes or other blood sugar-related illnesses should exercise care. Apple cider vinegar may interfere with drugs or lead to unexpected changes in blood sugar levels.

4. Potassium Depletion

Some study shows that excessive drinking of apple cider vinegar may contribute to potassium depletion in the body. Individuals with pre-existing potassium imbalances or illnesses that need careful monitoring of potassium levels should visit a healthcare professional before taking apple cider vinegar.

5. Gastrointestinal Distress

In rare situations, ingesting significant doses of apple cider vinegar may produce gastrointestinal distress, diarrhea, or other digestive difficulties.

Starting with a lesser dose and gradually increasing it may help lessen this danger.

6. Interaction with Drugs

Apple cider vinegar may interfere with some drugs, including diuretics and treatments for diabetes and heart diseases. If you are using drugs, contact a healthcare practitioner before using apple cider vinegar to examine possible interactions.

7. Allergic Responses

While uncommon, some people may develop allergic responses to apple cider vinegar or its components. If you have a history of allergies to apples or other similar compounds, try testing a tiny quantity of diluted apple cider vinegar before regular use.

8. Individual Variability

It's vital to realize that individual reactions to apple cider vinegar might differ. Genetics, tolerance levels, and general health have a crucial effect on how your body responds.

Monitoring your body's reaction and regulating your usage appropriately is crucial.

By weighing the possible advantages of appetite suppression, blood sugar control, and metabolism support with the potential dangers of side effects, you empower yourself to make choices that line with your health objectives and desires which hopefully you'll do holistically.

Integrating Apple Cider Vinegar: Dosing Recommendations and Practical Tips

Incorporating apple cider vinegar into your daily routine demands a balanced strategy that incorporates dose guidelines and practical ideas for a smooth experience. As you continue on this adventure, here's a guide to help you make the most of apple cider vinegar's potential benefits:

1. **Dosing Recommendations**

- Starting dose: Begin with a moderate dose to analyze your body's reaction. A usual starting point is 1 to 2 teaspoons (5 to 10 milliliters) of apple cider vinegar diluted in a big glass of water.

- Gradual Increase: If well-tolerated, try gradually increasing the dose over time. For example, you may raise the dose to 1 to 2 tablespoons (15 to 30 milliliters) diluted in water.

- Daily Limit: It's typically suggested to restrict your daily usage to no more than 2 tablespoons (30 milliliters). Excessive use may raise the risk of possible adverse effects.

2. Dilution Techniques

- Water Dilution: Dilute apple cider vinegar in a big glass of water before ingestion. This helps lessen its acidity and minimizes the danger of stomach pain or dental enamel loss.

- Honey or Maple Syrup: For extra taste, you may sweeten your diluted apple cider vinegar with a tiny quantity of honey or maple syrup.

3. Timing Considerations

- Before Meals: Consuming apple cider vinegar before meals may aid with hunger management. Consider taking it 20 to 30 minutes before your big meals.

- Meal Replacement: Some people include apple cider vinegar into their daily routine by using it as a salad dressing or adding it to foods as a taste enhancer.

4. Frequency

- Everyday Consistency: For maximum effects, strive to drink apple cider vinegar every day. Consistency is crucial to seeing its potential advantages over time.

5. Adjusting to Your Tolerance

- Individual Variability: Keep in mind that individual reactions differ. Some individuals may be more sensitive to the flavor or acidity of apple cider vinegar. Adjust the dose and dilution procedure to meet your tolerance.

6. **Monitoring Your Body's Response**

- Self-Awareness: Pay attention to how your body reacts to apple cider vinegar. Note changes in digestion, energy levels, appetite, and general well-being.

7. **Professional Guidance**

- Existing Health disorders: If you have pre-existing health disorders, including diabetes, gastrointestinal troubles, or renal problems, visit a healthcare practitioner before introducing apple cider vinegar into your regimen.

8. **Potential Interactions**

- Drugs: Apple cider vinegar may interfere with some drugs. If you are taking medication, obtain advice from a healthcare expert to confirm compatibility.

Glucomannan

The Satiety Superstar for Weight Management

Glucomannan, a soluble fiber isolated from the konjac root, has earned notoriety for its amazing ability to enhance satiety and aid in weight reduction attempts.

Glucomannan's unique ability to induce satiety, delay stomach emptying, and regulate blood sugar levels makes a strong argument for its inclusion in the arsenal of natural supplements for weight control. By introducing this soluble fiber into your routine, you tap into a mechanism that allows you to make thoughtful nutritional choices and begin on a sustained road toward reaching and maintaining a healthy weight.

As we look into the methods via which glucomannan exerts its benefits, the power of this natural supplement in helping weight control becomes evident:

1. The Power of Soluble Fiber

Glucomannan belongs to the group of soluble fibers—substances that absorb water and produce a thick gel-like consistency in the digestive system. This particular feature serves as the basis for its involvement in increasing satiety and assisting weight reduction.

2. Enhanced Satiety and Fullness

When taken, glucomannan absorbs water in the stomach and expands, giving a sensation of fullness and satiety. This physical enlargement stimulates receptors in the stomach lining, delivering messages to the brain that express the experience of fullness. As a consequence, people may feel satiated with fewer quantities of food, resulting in lower calorie consumption.

3. Delayed Gastric Emptying

Glucomannan's gel-like nature leads to delayed gastric emptying—the process by which food exits the stomach and enters the small intestine. This delay prolongs the length of fullness and minimizes the frequency of hunger sensations, making it simpler to adhere to restricted eating habits.

4. Blood Sugar Regulation

Soluble fibers like glucomannan also have a role in balancing blood sugar levels. The gel generated by glucomannan slows down the absorption of sugars and carbs from the digestive system into the circulation. This leads to a slow increase and fall in blood sugar levels, eliminating sudden spikes and crashes that might induce cravings.

5. Impact on Gut Microbiota

Emerging research shows that glucomannan's fermentation in the colon by beneficial gut bacteria may contribute to enhanced gut health. A healthy gut microbiota has been related to weight control, and glucomannan's possible function in fostering a balanced gut environment adds to its overall advantages.

6. Reduction in calorie consumption

By encouraging feelings of fullness and lowering hunger, glucomannan may naturally lead to a reduction in total calorie consumption. This reduction in calories, when paired with a balanced diet and regular physical exercise, may lead to weight loss over time.

How Glucomannan Works in the Stomach

The amazing capacity of glucomannan to absorb water and expand inside the stomach is a critical aspect of its involvement in increasing satiety and helping weight reduction. Let's go into the mechanics of how this process unfolds:

1. **Unique Structure of Glucomannan**

Glucomannan is a soluble fiber defined by its structure of long chains of glucose and mannose molecules. This structure enables it to create a gel-like material when it comes into touch with water.

2. **Absorption of Water**

Upon intake, glucomannan enters the stomach in its dry and granular state. As it enters the acidic environment of the stomach, it immediately starts to absorb water. This absorption is a consequence of the hydrophilic (water-attracting) characteristic of the fiber's molecular structure.

3. **Formation of Viscous Gel**

As glucomannan absorbs water, it turns into a very viscous and gel-like material. This gel creates a thick matrix inside the stomach, occupying a large volume.

4. **Signals to Satiety Receptors**

The physical presence of the gel generated by glucomannan activates receptors inside the stomach lining and the surrounding tissues. These receptors are crucial for communicating sensations of fullness and satisfaction to the brain.

5. Prolonged Satiety and Appetite Reduction

The expansion of the gel leads to a sensation of fullness and satiety, establishing a barrier that slows down the emptying of the stomach. This leads to an extended length of fullness, lowering the frequency of hunger signals and the impulse to eat.

6. Regulated Eating Behaviors

The extended satiety generated by glucomannan's gel-like nature aids regulated eating behaviors. Individuals may naturally eat smaller amounts and have lower calorie consumption as a consequence.

7. Gradual Absorption of Nutrients

The gel's presence in the stomach also affects the pace at which nutrients are delivered into the small intestine. This slow release may help to regulate blood sugar levels, reducing fast spikes and crashes that lead to cravings.

Potential Side Effects of Glucomannan

While glucomannan has potential advantages for boosting satiety and weight control, it's crucial to be aware of certain adverse effects that may emerge from its ingestion. As you study the introduction of glucomannan into your health regimen, here's a complete summary of the possible considerations:

1. Gastrointestinal Disturbances

Glucomannan's capacity to expand and create a gel-like material inside the stomach may cause gastrointestinal discomfort in certain persons. Bloating, gas, and stomach cramps are possible adverse effects that may develop, especially if glucomannan is not eaten with appropriate water.

2. **Difficulty Swallowing**

Glucomannan supplements are generally available in pill or tablet forms. For certain people, these capsules may enlarge in the throat before reaching the stomach, leading to a sense of difficulty swallowing. Ensuring proper water intake while using glucomannan capsules might help decrease this risk.

3. **Obstruction of the Esophagus**

In rare circumstances, ingestion of glucomannan without appropriate water intake may lead to the growth of the fiber in the esophagus, possibly creating a blockage. To avoid this, always take glucomannan supplements with a full glass of water.

4. Impact on drugs: Glucomannan's gel-like nature has the potential to impede the absorption of drugs taken concurrently. This may affect the efficacy of some drugs. To minimize interference, try taking drugs at a different time from glucomannan ingestion.

5. Choking danger: For persons who have trouble swallowing or who are prone to choking, glucomannan supplements may offer a choking danger, particularly if not taken with adequate water.

6. Interaction with Medical Problems: Individuals with certain medical problems, such as gastrointestinal disorders, should see a healthcare professional before taking glucomannan supplements. The gel-like material generated by glucomannan may worsen some gastrointestinal disorders.

7. Potential Allergic responses: While uncommon, some people may suffer allergic responses to glucomannan or other components found in supplements. If you have a history of allergies, try testing a tiny quantity of glucomannan before regular ingestion.

Dosages, Timing, and Optimal Usage of Glucomannan

Incorporating glucomannan supplements into your weight control routine demands a strategic strategy that includes doses, timing, and correct administration. By sticking to these instructions, you may get the most of glucomannan's potential advantages while ensuring a safe and successful experience:

1. **Dosage Recommendations**

- Starting dose: Begin with a lesser dose and gradually raise it to analyze your body's reaction. A normal initial dose is roughly 1 gram (1,000 milligrams) taken with lots of water.

- Gradual Increase: If well-tolerated, try increasing the dose over time. Some people may ultimately eat up to 2 to 4 grams of glucomannan per day, split into many doses.

2. **Timing Considerations**

- Before Meals: To enhance the satiety-enhancing benefits, ingest glucomannan supplements roughly 15 to 30 minutes before meals. This timing permits the gel-like material to develop in the stomach and generate a sensation of fullness.

- Dose Division: If taking numerous doses throughout the day, strive to take them before each big meal to maintain regulated eating behaviors.

3. **Proper Usage**

- Hydration is Key: To minimize any negative effects and promote the safe expansion of glucomannan in the stomach, always take supplements with a full glass of water. This helps the fiber absorb water and form a gel-like consistency.

- Capsule or Powder Form: Glucomannan supplements are available in capsule or powder form. If taking capsules, ensure you drink adequate water to help in swallowing and avoid any choking danger.

4. Individual Tolerance

- Self-Monitoring: Pay careful attention to how your body reacts to glucomannan supplementation. Note any changes in digestion, fullness, and general well-being.

- Altering dose: If you suffer stomach discomfort or other negative effects, try lowering the dose or altering your intake methods.

5. Interaction with Medications

- Medication Timing: If you use medicines, ensure there is a time interval between medication intake and glucomannan administration. The gel-like material generated by glucomannan may alter the absorption of medicines.

6. Consultation with Healthcare Provider

- Existing Health concerns: If you have pre-existing health concerns or are on medication, see a healthcare practitioner before introducing glucomannan supplements into your regimen.

This strategy enables you to leverage the power of this soluble fiber to boost satiety, regulate eating, and eventually contribute to your overall weight management objectives.

Individual Considerations for Supplement Integration

As we've gone through the realm of natural supplements for weight loss, it's crucial to stop and think about the value of uniqueness in your approach. Your wellness path is uniquely yours, molded by your requirements, objectives, and health state. Here, we invite you to adopt an attitude of empowerment, individualized choices, and conscious integration as you investigate the possible advantages of various supplements.

1. **Your Health Narrative**

The cornerstone of a successful supplement integration lies in a comprehensive grasp of your health narrative. Each individual's health state is diverse, determined by variables such as medical history, present ailments, and medicines. Before making any adjustments, discussing your healthcare practitioner ensures that your decisions are in accordance with your health requirements.

2. **Defining Your Goals**

Set clear objectives for your health journey. Are you seeking appetite management, metabolism assistance, or greater energy? By identifying your objectives, you develop a plan that corresponds with your desires.

3. Mindful Choices: When purchasing supplements, focus on quality over quantity.

Research brands, study labels, and choose credible suppliers that stress transparency and purity.

4. Acknowledging Individual Variability

Just as no two persons are alike, reactions to supplements might differ. Genetics, lifestyle, and current health concerns all have a role in how your body reacts to these chemicals. Be patient and sensitive to your body's cues.

5. Integrating Holistically

Supplements are tools within a greater health toolset. They function best when supported with a balanced diet, frequent exercise, stress management, and adequate sleep.

6. Monitoring and Adaptation

As you incorporate supplements, pay attention to your body's reactions. Adjust doses, timing, or even the supplements themselves if required. This adaptable strategy guarantees that your trip stays dynamic and sensitive to your demands.

7. **Sustainable Decisions**

Consider the sustainability of your decisions. Focus on building a lifestyle that promotes your well-being for the long term rather than chasing fast cures.

8. **Mind-Body Connection**

Your body frequently expresses its wants and reactions. Tune into your intuition and heed the messages it sends.

CHAPTER 3

Integrating Supplements into a Healthy Lifestyle

The Role of Balanced Nutrition

A balanced diet, physical exercise, and mental well-being are the pillars of a comprehensive and sustainable approach to health and wellbeing. These three pillars operate in unison to promote total well-being and should be the cornerstone of any healthy lifestyle:

1. Balanced Nutrition

Important Nutrients: A balanced diet supplies the body with important nutrients, including vitamins, minerals, protein, carbs, and healthy fats, required for optimum functioning.

Energy Balance: Maintaining a balance between the calories ingested and expended is vital for maintaining weight and avoiding chronic illnesses.

Diverse Diet: A diversified and diverse diet ensures that the body obtains a broad variety of nutrients, supporting general health and lowering the chance of nutritional shortages.

Hydration: Proper hydration is crucial for digestion, circulation, temperature control, and general vigor.

2. Physical Activity

Cardiovascular Health: Regular physical exercise strengthens the heart, improves circulation, and minimizes the risk of cardiovascular disorders.

Weight Management: Exercise plays a significant part in obtaining and maintaining a healthy weight by boosting calorie expenditure and creating lean muscle.

Mental Health: Physical exercise generates endorphins, which may decrease stress, anxiety, and symptoms of depression, leading to enhanced mental well-being.

Bone and Muscular Health: Weight-bearing workouts assist in preserving bone density and muscular mass, especially crucial as we age.

Quality of Life: An active lifestyle promotes mobility, flexibility, and general quality of life by boosting functional fitness.

3. **Mental Well-Being**

Stress Management: Techniques like meditation, mindfulness, and relaxation techniques assist in managing stress, lowering its influence on physical and mental health.

Emotional Resilience: Strong mental well-being creates emotional resilience, helping people to deal with life's adversities more successfully.

Social Connection: Building and sustaining connections and a solid support network favorably improve mental health.

Cognitive Function: Mental well-being is related to greater cognitive function, memory, and decision-making ability.

Sleep: Quality sleep is vital for mental well-being since it improves mood control and cognitive performance.

While natural supplements may play a crucial role in addressing particular health requirements, they should be considered complementary to these three core pillars.

Understanding the Synergy

Natural supplements may complement a healthy lifestyle by supplying extra nutrients, supporting particular health objectives, and addressing any nutritional shortages. Here's how they can function in harmony with a healthy lifestyle:

1. Filling Nutrient Gaps

Even with a well-balanced diet, it may be tough to receive all the critical vitamins, minerals, and other elements required for good health. Natural supplements may help cover these vitamin gaps, ensuring the body obtains the required components for numerous physical activities.

2. Supporting Specific Health Goals

Natural supplements may be designed to assist specific health goals. For instance, those trying to strengthen their immune system would take vitamin C and zinc supplements, while those looking to promote joint health might choose glucosamine and chondroitin. These supplements may give focused assistance in addition to a balanced diet.

3. Enhancing Nutrient Absorption

Some supplements, such as probiotics and digestive enzymes, may boost nutrient absorption by supporting healthy gut flora and optimizing digestion. This may optimize the advantages of the nutrients gained from diet.

4. Balancing Deficiencies

In circumstances when people have detected nutritional deficiencies via medical testing, natural supplements may serve as a focused strategy to remedy these imbalances. This is typically advised under the advice of a healthcare practitioner.

5. Promoting Overall Wellness

Supplements containing antioxidants, such as vitamin E or resveratrol, may help counteract oxidative stress and lower the risk of chronic illnesses. This supports a healthy lifestyle's emphasis on illness prevention.

6. Aiding in Weight Management

Some natural supplements, as discussed previously, may help weight management efforts by improving metabolism, decreasing hunger, or stimulating fat loss. When taken in combination with a balanced diet and moderate exercise, they may boost the efficacy of weight control measures.

7. Stress Reduction and Mental Well-Being

Adaptogenic herbs such as ashwagandha and ginseng may help the body adapt to stress and improve emotional well-being. They may support stress management approaches like meditation or yoga.

8. Athletic Performance and Recovery

Supplements including branched-chain amino acids (BCAAs) and creatine may enhance muscle development, increase exercise performance, and help in post-workout recovery. Athletes and fitness enthusiasts might benefit from these substances when included in their regimens.

9. Supporting Special Dietary Needs

Individuals with dietary restrictions or specialized diets (e.g., vegetarian, vegan) may benefit from supplements that assist in addressing any nutritional deficits linked with their dietary choices, such as vitamin B12 for vegetarians.

10. Optimizing Aging Health

As people age, some nutritional needs may vary. Supplements like calcium and vitamin D become increasingly necessary for bone health, while CoQ10 may improve cardiovascular health. Supplements suited to age-related requirements may boost general well-being.

It's vital to underline that natural supplements are supposed to "supplement" a healthy lifestyle, not replace it. They function most successfully when taken in combination with a balanced diet, regular exercise, proper sleep, stress management, and other good practices.

How might supplements target particular dietary deficits or assist metabolic functions?

Balanced nutrition is the cornerstone of well-being, supplying the body with critical nutrients for energy, repair, and general vitality.

However, amid the hustle and bustle of contemporary life, it's not unusual to have nutritional gaps in our diet. This is when natural supplements come in as useful companions.

Addressing Nutritional Gaps

Supplements are meant to replace certain nutritional gaps that may emerge due to dietary choices, constraints, or lifestyle circumstances. For instance, if your diet lacks appropriate quantities of a certain vitamin, mineral, or amino acid, a specialized supplement may guarantee you achieve your daily needs.

This supplement is not designed to replace entire foods but to complement them, offering a safety net for optimum health.

Metabolic Support

Our metabolism, the complex chain of chemical processes that maintain life, plays a vital role in weight regulation. Metabolic processes transform food into energy, and how effectively this occurs varies from person to person. Natural supplements may support and enhance metabolic functioning in numerous ways:

1. Enhancing Energy Synthesis

Certain supplements, such as B vitamins and Coenzyme Q10, are involved in energy synthesis inside cells. Ensuring an appropriate intake of these nutrients may promote metabolic efficiency, perhaps leading to better energy levels and calorie usage.

2. Regulating Blood Sugar

Chromium and alpha-lipoic acid are supplements recognized for their involvement in regulating blood sugar levels. By boosting insulin sensitivity, they may help control appetite and minimize cravings, leading to weight management.

3. **Supporting Thyroid Function**

Iodine, selenium, and zinc are key elements for thyroid health. A well-functioning thyroid is vital for controlling metabolism. Supplements containing these minerals may assist in thyroid function and overall metabolic balance.

4. **Promoting Fat Utilization**

Some supplements, such as green tea extract and conjugated linoleic acid (CLA), are known to promote fat metabolism. While not a replacement for exercise and a balanced diet, they may aid in the usage of stored fat for energy.

It's crucial to remember that the efficacy of supplements in addressing nutritional shortages and aiding metabolism might differ from person to person. The choice to integrate supplements should be made in cooperation with a healthcare practitioner who can analyze your unique requirements and propose acceptable solutions.

In summary, supplements serve a significant role in resolving dietary shortages and supporting metabolic activities. When incorporated into a comprehensive strategy that includes a balanced diet, physical exercise, and mental well-being, they become crucial tools in your path toward sustainable weight control and general health.

Practical Tips for Integration: Scheduling Supplement Intake

While integrating natural supplements into your daily routine, one of the primary obstacles is ensuring that their consumption doesn't disturb your life but instead becomes a seamless part of your health path. Here are ideas to help you arrange supplement usage without disruption:

1. **Consistency is Key**
Choose a certain time each day to take your vitamins. Consistency strengthens the habit and decreases the probability of forgetting.

2. Align with Meals

Many supplements are better absorbed when taken with meals. Consider taking them with a meal, which also assists in linking supplement use with regular mealtimes.

3. Use a Pill Organizer

Invest in a pill organizer with daily slots. Fill it for the week or month ahead, making it simple to keep track of your supplement program.

4. Set Reminders

Use smartphone alarms or reminders to stimulate your supplement consumption at the scheduled time. Apps developed for medication reminders may be especially beneficial.

5. Create Visual Cues

Place your supplement bottles or organizer in a conspicuous position, such as near to your toothbrush or coffee machine. This acts as a visual indication of your everyday activity.

6. Pair with Existing Habits

Pair supplement consumption with an existing habit or activity, such as your morning coffee or nightly beauty regimen. This way, it becomes a normal part of your day.

7. Divide the Dose

If a supplement takes many doses per day, divide them carefully. For instance, if a dosage is prescribed with breakfast and supper, you may take one at breakfast and the other with your evening meal.

8. Travel-Friendly Solutions

When traveling or on the road, utilize travel-sized pill containers or pre-packaged dosages to continue your supplement program without interruption.

9. Consult a Healthcare Practitioner

Seek help from a healthcare practitioner to identify the ideal time for certain supplements, especially if you're taking prescription drugs.

10. Keep a Record

Maintain a supplement record to chronicle your consumption, any noticed effects, and any modifications made. This helps you keep organized and informed.

11. Be Mindful of Interactions

Understand possible interactions between supplements and between supplements and meals or drugs. Consult with a healthcare practitioner to check compatibility.

12. Stay Hydrated

Drink a proper quantity of water while taking supplements to aid with digestion and absorption. However, certain supplements may need to be taken with minimum water to prevent dilution.

13. Follow Prescribed Doses

Read the label carefully and follow the prescribed doses and directions supplied by the manufacturer or your healthcare provider. Avoid exceeding the prescribed consumption, since this might lead to harmful consequences.

14. Quality Matters

Choose reputed brands and high-quality supplements. Look for third-party testing and certification to assure purity and efficacy. Your healthcare practitioner may suggest reputable brands.

15. Adjust your Lifestyle Changes

If your lifestyle or dietary habits change (e.g., you start a new diet or exercise program), evaluate your supplement regimen with your healthcare professional to ensure it stays suitable.

16. Regularly Evaluate Your Regimen

Periodically evaluate your supplement regimen with your healthcare physician. Needs might alter over time, and you may need to modify your supplements appropriately.

17. Storage Matters

Store supplements in a cool, dry area away from direct sunlight and moisture. Keep them out of reach of minors.

18. **Be Patient**

Supplements may take time to generate significant results. Be patient and reasonable in your aspirations. Results vary based on individual characteristics and the supplement's intended function.

19. **Do Not Self-Diagnose**

Avoid self-diagnosing health concerns and taking supplements as a substitute for medical therapy. Always visit a healthcare expert for an appropriate diagnosis and treatment plan.

Everyone's schedule is unique, so adjust these tactics to fit your lifestyle and tastes. The objective is to make supplement ingestion an easy and integral part of your everyday life, supporting your holistic health path without disturbance.

Synergy between Food Choices and Effectiveness

The synergy between dietary choices and the efficacy of weight loss pills is a vital aspect of your route to reaching your health and fitness objectives. Here, we look into the fundamental link between what you consume and how your body reacts to substances marketed to assist in weight loss:

1. **Nutrient Absorption**

Your food choices substantially determine how efficiently your body absorbs nutrients from weight loss supplements.

Some supplements function more efficiently when taken with particular kinds of foods. For example, fat-soluble vitamins, typically included in weight reduction aids, are absorbed better when ingested with dietary fats.

2. **Whole Foods vs. Isolated Nutrients**

Whole foods contain a variety of nutrients, fiber, and phytochemicals that synergistically help weight reduction.

Weight reduction pills, although targeted, frequently deliver isolated nutrients. For a comprehensive strategy, include healthy meals that naturally help your weight reduction quest.

3. Balanced Diets Enhance Supplement Effectiveness

A balanced diet that comprises nutrient-dense meals creates a good basis for the efficiency of weight reduction pills. These supplements may thus operate as targeted enhancers, addressing particular demands within your larger dietary choices.

4. Food Interactions

Be conscious of how your food choices may interact with weight loss products. For example, caffeine-containing supplements might affect your sleep, so it's recommended to timing their consumption carefully. Consulting a healthcare expert may help you through these exchanges.

5. Personalized Approach

Weight loss is a very personal process. Your eating habits, nutritional needs, and weight reduction objectives should drive your supplement selections.

6. Food Sources of Nutrients

Remember that weight reduction pills are meant to complement, not replace, the nutrients contained in entire meals.

Whenever feasible, aim for meals rich in the vitamins and minerals that help weight reduction. For instance, if you're aiming to improve your fiber intake for satiety, consider whole grains, legumes, and fruits.

7. Balanced Nutrition as the Foundation

The efficacy of weight reduction supplements is most obvious when they are incorporated into a balanced and nutrient-rich diet suited for weight control. Supplements should be considered as helpful tools within the larger context of your dietary choices.

The interaction between dietary choices and the efficacy of weight loss supplements is vital on your way to attaining your weight reduction objectives. A diet rich in nutrient-dense, complete foods provides the best background for weight reduction pills to be most successful. These supplements are great partners, serving particular demands while whole foods give a larger variety of nutrients and advantages. Tailor your food choices and supplement usage to maximize their synergy on your weight reduction journey.

Foods that are naturally high in Minerals found in Supplements

One key component of your weight reduction journey is exploiting the synergy between food choices and weight loss supplements. Here, we'll investigate some foods that are naturally high in the same nutrients typically found in supplements meant to promote weight loss:

1. Fiber-Rich Foods

Fruits and Vegetables: These nutritious powerhouses are rich with dietary fiber, a nutrient that promotes a sensation of fullness and helps regulate hunger. Fiber also aids healthy digestion. Incorporate a range of bright fruits and leafy greens into your regular diet.

2. Protein Sources

Lean Meats: Skinless chicken, lean cuts of beef, and fish are good sources of lean protein. Protein assists with muscle maintenance and adds to a sensation of fullness, lowering the temptation to overeat.

Legumes: Beans, lentils, and chickpeas give plant-based protein coupled with fiber, making them a beneficial addition to weight reduction regimens.

3. **Healthy Fats**

Avocado: Rich in monounsaturated fats, avocados are a heart-healthy alternative that also delivers a delightful creamy texture to dishes.

Fatty Fish: Salmon, mackerel, and sardines are strong in omega-3 fatty acids, believed to enhance general health and perhaps assist in weight reduction.

4. **Calcium Sources**

Dairy Products: Low-fat or Greek yogurt, milk, and cheese are calcium-rich meals that also deliver protein. Calcium has a part in metabolic processes and may aid in weight control.

Leafy Greens: Broccoli, kale, and spinach are non-dairy sources of calcium.

5. **Green Tea**

Green tea is naturally abundant in antioxidants called catechins, which are considered to increase metabolism and help weight reduction. Enjoy a cup of green tea as a pleasant beverage.

6. **Whole Grains**

Oats: Rolled oats are a source of soluble fiber known as beta-glucan, which may help lower hunger and increase fullness.

Quinoa: This whole grain is not only high in fiber but also offers a full source of protein.

7. **Spices and Herbs**

Cayenne Pepper: The chemical capsaicin in cayenne pepper may have a thermogenic effect, possibly enhancing calorie burning.

Cinnamon: Cinnamon is known to help balance blood sugar levels, lowering cravings for sweet meals.

8. **Nuts and Seeds**

Almonds: These nuts are a source of healthful fats, protein, and fiber. A little handful of almonds may be a fulfilling snack that suppresses hunger.

9. **Berries**

Blueberries, Strawberries, Raspberries: Berries are low in calories and rich in antioxidants and fiber. They're a fantastic way to satisfy sweet cravings while boosting satiety.

10. **Chia Seeds**

These small seeds are rich in fiber, which swells in the stomach, helping to suppress hunger and induce a sensation of fullness.

11. **Eggs**

Eggs are a source of high-quality protein, and the protein in eggs may help you feel full and satisfied.

12. **Grapefruit**

This citrus fruit is renowned for its ability to boost weight reduction, potentially owing to components that help control blood sugar and lower insulin levels.

13. **Lean Turkey**

Like chicken, turkey is a lean source of protein that may help you feel full and promote muscle maintenance.

14. Beans

Along with protein, beans are high in fiber, making them a full and healthful addition to salads, soups, and entrees.

15. Nuts & Seeds (2)

Walnuts: Walnuts are not only a source of healthy fats but also contain omega-3 fatty acids, which may have extra advantages for weight control.

These foods, rich in nutrients typically found in weight reduction pills, provide a broad and delicious variety of alternatives for your weight loss quest.

Incorporating these items into your diet not only supplies important nutrients but also corresponds with the very nutrients commonly found in weight reduction products. The mix of complete, natural meals with specific supplements gives a holistic approach to attaining your weight reduction objectives.

The Role of Exercise in Amplifying Supplement Effects

Most of us don't want any stress, or love the pains that come with exercising, some have no time because of the amount of time they need to spend on work, studies etcetera.

While weight loss supplements can offer valuable support in your journey toward a healthier you, their effectiveness can be significantly amplified when combined with regular exercise, no matter how little. Here's how exercise synergizes with supplements to enhance their benefits:

1. **Metabolic Boost**

Exercise, particularly high-intensity interval training (HIIT) and strength training may rev up your metabolism.

This higher metabolic rate means your body burns more calories, possibly improving the weight reduction benefits of supplements.

2. **Muscle Maintenance and Development**

Supplements like protein and branched-chain amino acids (BCAAs) may assist in muscle maintenance and development. When you participate in resistance training or strength exercises, these supplements become even more helpful by giving your muscles the required building blocks for strength and tone.

3. **Hunger Regulation**

Exercise may help manage hunger by altering hormones like ghrelin and leptin. When hunger is well managed, you're more likely to stick to your food plan and supplement routine.

4. **Enhanced Nutrient Delivery**

Exercise enhances blood flow and nutrient delivery to your cells. This implies that the nutrients in your supplements are carried more effectively to where they're required, improving their efficacy.

5. Stress Reduction

Regular physical exercise is a recognized stress reducer. By reducing stress levels, exercise complements nutrients that improve mental well-being, providing a pleasant atmosphere for weight reduction.

6. Improved Insulin Sensitivity

Aerobic activity, such as vigorous walking or running, might enhance insulin sensitivity. This means your body uses blood sugar more efficiently, perhaps lowering sugar cravings and assisting in weight control.

7. Fat Utilization

Certain supplements, such as green tea extract and conjugated linoleic acid (CLA), are known to improve fat metabolism. When paired with aerobic activities, these supplements may further improve the use of stored fat for energy.

8. Consistency and Long-Term Success

Regular exercise creates discipline and consistency. By adopting a program that involves both exercise and supplement use, you're more likely to continue your weight reduction efforts in the long run.

9. Mental Resilience

Exercise is not just a physical struggle but also a mental one. It increases mental toughness and tenacity, which may be useful while tackling the ups and downs of a weight reduction journey.

10. General Well-Being

Exercise adds to general physical and emotional well-being, establishing a positive feedback loop with supplements targeted to assist weight reduction and holistic health.

Types of Exercises that Synergize with Supplements for Weight Loss

When it comes to enhancing the benefits of weight reduction pills, picking the correct sorts of activities is crucial. Here are insights on activities that nicely fit with supplement usage:

1. Cardiovascular Exercises

Aerobic Workouts: Activities like brisk walking, running, cycling, and swimming are fantastic for burning calories and boosting cardiovascular fitness. They correlate well with weight reduction pills by raising calorie expenditure, possibly magnifying the benefits of fat-burning supplements.

2. High-Intensity Interval Training (HIIT)

HIIT comprises short bursts of intensive activity followed by shorter recuperation intervals. This sort of exercise may be very beneficial in improving metabolism and promoting fat burning. It combines nicely with substances meant to boost calorie and fat metabolism.

3. **Strength Training**

Resistance Exercises: Strength training, including weight lifting and bodyweight movements, helps develop and maintain lean muscle mass. Supplements like protein and BCAAs are useful here, promoting muscle rehabilitation and development. Muscle burns more calories at rest, aiding weight control.

4. **Flexibility and Balance**

Yoga and Pilates: These workouts concentrate on flexibility, balance, and core strength. While not powerful calorie burners, they boost general well-being. Supplements encouraging stress reduction and mental well-being match well with these workouts.

5. **Mind-Body Practices**

Tai Chi and Qigong: These moderate, contemplative techniques increase balance, mental attention, and general vigor. They correlate with vitamins that help stress management and overall well-being.

6. Consistency and Variety

Consistency is crucial to long-term success. Choose workouts you love and can commit to consistently. Variety in your workout program keeps things exciting and avoids plateaus in your weight reduction quest.

7. Lifestyle Incorporation

Look for chances to keep active throughout the day. Simple behaviors like taking the stairs instead of the elevator or walking during breaks might complement supplement consumption by adding to calorie expenditure.

8. Personalization

The choice of workouts should coincide with your weight reduction objectives and fitness level. Consult with a fitness expert to design a specific workout plan that compliments your supplement regimen.

9. Hydration (Stay Hydrated)

Regardless of the sort of activity you do, proper hydration is vital. Supplements, particularly those in powdered form, may need higher fluid consumption to guarantee their efficiency.

Remember that the efficacy of exercise and supplements differs from person to person. It's crucial to listen to your body, be consistent, and seek help from a healthcare practitioner or fitness expert when incorporating vitamins and exercise into your weight reduction approach. When paired wisely, vitamins and exercise become effective tools in your quest for a healthier and fitter self.

Mind-Body Connection: The Vital Role of Mental Well-Being in Weight Loss

In the goal of weight reduction and general well-being, the relevance of mental well-being cannot be emphasized. Here, we explain why a pleasant mental state is a cornerstone of success in your weight reduction journey:

1. **Mind-Body Connection**

Mental well-being is directly tied to your physical health. Stress, worry, and negative emotions may promote unhealthy eating behaviors and impair your weight reduction success. Supplements that promote stress reduction and mood control may be important allies.

2. **Emotional Eating Awareness**

Emotional eating, frequently motivated by stress or negative emotions, may undermine even the most meticulously planned diets. Cultivating mental resilience and employing supplements that address emotional well-being will help you break away from this pattern.

3. **Long-Term Commitment**

Weight reduction is a process, not a destination. Mental well-being creates the patience and drive required for long-term success. Supplements that promote cognitive function and mental clarity might assist in making educated decisions along your trip.

4. Self-Image and Self-Care

A healthy self-image is intricately related to mental well-being. When you feel good about yourself, you're more likely to participate in self-care behaviors that coincide with your weight reduction objectives. Supplements meant to improve self-esteem and confidence may play a role here.

5. Resilience to Setbacks

Weight reduction typically entails plateaus and setbacks. A robust mental approach helps you overcome these hurdles without losing sight of your ultimate aim. Supplements that enhance mental resilience and flexibility may be useful.

6. Goal Defining and Motivation

Mental well-being plays a crucial role in defining realistic objectives and remaining motivated. Supplements that boost attention and motivation might assist in sustaining the drive required to attain your targeted results.

7. **Reducing Stress-Induced Weight Increase**
Chronic stress may lead to weight increase owing to hormonal changes that alter appetite and fat storage. Stress-reduction pills may attenuate these effects, producing a more favorable environment for weight loss.

8. **Lifestyle Enjoyment**
A pleasant and optimistic mentality promotes a passion for lifestyle adjustments that help weight reduction. Supplements may complement this by enhancing emotions of satisfaction and happiness.

9. **Expert Support**
Mental well-being typically benefits from expert assistance. Consulting with a therapist, counselor, or coach may give skills for managing stress, emotions, and self-esteem throughout your weight reduction journey.

Mental well-being is not merely a supporting component in your weight reduction journey; it is a core essential. A healthy mind prepares the path for effective weight control by minimizing mental obstacles, boosting resilience, and fostering self-care.

Supplements that target different elements of mental well-being will be important aids in obtaining and keeping your weight reduction objectives.

Mindfulness and Stress Reduction: Tools for Weight Loss Success

In your weight loss journey, establishing mental well-being is frequently as crucial as food choices and exercise. Incorporating mindfulness practices and stress reduction approaches may substantially contribute to your success. Here are some successful strategies:

1. Mindful Eating

Practice Mindful Eating: Paying complete attention to your meals helps decrease overeating. Savor each meal, chew gently, and engage your senses. This activity promotes awareness of hunger and fullness signals, supporting healthy eating behaviors.

2. Mindfulness Meditation

Regular meditation sessions help decrease stress and emotional eating. Dedicate a few minutes every day to concentrate on your breath, thoughts, and physiological sensations. This cultivates consciousness, helping you to make thoughtful dietary choices.

3. Yoga for Stress Reduction

Yoga incorporates physical postures, breathing exercises, and meditation. It relieves tension, increases flexibility, and boosts body awareness. Yoga may be a peaceful supplement to your weight reduction quest.

4. Deep Breathing Exercises

When stress levels rise, take a minute to practice deep breathing. Inhale deeply for a count of four, hold for four, and exhale for four. Repeat numerous times to soothe the nervous system.

5. Visualization

Positive Visualization: Visualize your weight reduction objectives and the strategies to accomplish them. This positive visualization may enhance motivation and provide a feeling of success.

6. Progressive Muscle Relaxation

This method includes tensing and then relaxing muscle groups systematically. It helps reduce bodily tension and is very useful for stress relief.

7. Effective Time Management

Organize your daily agenda to incorporate rest and self-care. Balancing your schedule minimizes the stress associated with a hurried existence.

8. Gratitude Practice

Gratitude Journaling: Write down things you're thankful for every day. Shifting your emphasis to pleasant parts of life may decrease stress and increase mental well-being.

9. Social Support

Connect with Supportive Individuals: Share your weight reduction journey with friends, family, or a support group. Talking about your problems and triumphs helps decrease tension.

10. Mindful Movement (Walking Meditation)

Combine mindfulness and physical exercise by practicing walking meditation. Pay attention to each step and your surroundings while you walk, creating mental clarity and calm.

11. Professional Guidance

Therapy or Counseling: If stress severely inhibits your weight reduction success, consider receiving help from a therapist or counselor. They may give individualized solutions for controlling stress and emotional well-being.

You should have it in mind that the efficiency of these strategies may vary from person to person. Experiment with various techniques to discover ones that connect with you and boost your mental well-being. Combining these mindfulness and stress reduction strategies with vitamins meant to boost mental health will help build a sturdy foundation for your weight loss journey.

Navigating Challenges: Weight Loss Challenges

As women, we face unique challenges when it comes to achieving holistic well-being. But don't worry, you're not alone. There are practical strategies you can use to overcome these obstacles and empower yourself.

Let's take a look at some common hurdles and how to navigate them with empathy and self-care:

1. Hormonal Shifts

Our bodies are constantly changing, and that's okay. It's important to find supplements that work for your specific needs during different phases and to seek personalized advice from healthcare professionals.

2. Metabolic Realities

Quick fixes are tempting, but sustainable lifestyle changes are better for your overall well-being. Focus on a mix of cardiovascular and strength-training exercises and choose supplements that support your metabolism and energy levels.

3. Social Pressures

It's time to redefine beauty on your own terms. Surround yourself with positive influences and seek support from like-minded communities. Remember to celebrate your body's strength and resilience.

4. Emotional Eating

We all have emotional triggers, but it's important to develop awareness and cultivate alternative coping mechanisms such as mindfulness and journaling. Choose supplements that promote emotional well-being.

5. **Positive Body Image**

Practicing self-love and gratitude for your body is crucial. Engage in activities that make you feel strong and capable, and use supplements as enhancers rather than measures to conform to external standards.

6. **Balanced Diet**

Prioritizing a diverse and balanced diet is key. Identify nutritional gaps and consult a nutritionist for personalized guidance on supplementing your diet effectively.

7. **Mental Health**

Integrating stress-reducing practices such as meditation is essential. Remember to seek professional help when needed and choose supplements that support cognitive function and emotional well-being.

8. Sorting Through Information Overload

It can be overwhelming to navigate the supplement landscape but don't worry. Rely on reputable sources and consult healthcare professionals for guidance on supplement choices.

9. Fitness Expectations

It's important to set realistic fitness goals and find joy in movement. Supplements can aid recovery and energy levels as you engage in physical activity.

10. Realistic Expectations

Remember to celebrate small victories and progress, and set achievable milestones. Use supplements to support, not replace, your efforts toward long-term well-being.

Remember, progress takes time. But with empathy and self-care, you can overcome these challenges and achieve holistic well-being. Don't be afraid to seek personalized advice when needed, and always prioritize your well-being.

Strategies for Overcoming Hurdles in Supplement Integration

Integrating vitamins into your weight reduction journey may be tremendously useful, but it's not necessarily without its problems. Here are some ideas to assist you in overcoming typical hurdles:

1. See a Healthcare Practitioner

If you're unclear about whether supplements are best for you or if you have underlying health issues, see a healthcare practitioner. They may give tailored advice and ensure your supplement selections are safe and effective.

2. Create a Routine

Consistency is crucial with supplements. Establish a regular schedule for taking them, such as with meals or at a certain time each day. This practice makes it easy to remember and lowers the likelihood of skipping doses.

3. **Read Labels Carefully**

Understanding what's in your supplements is vital. Read labels to verify you're receiving the ingredients you need and that the product satisfies quality requirements. Look for certificates from recognized organizations.

4. **Start Slowly**

When introducing new supplements, start with one at a time to observe how your body reacts. This helps detect any bad reactions or sensitivities.

5. **Stay Hydrated**

Some supplements may need increased fluid intake for maximum absorption. Ensure you keep well-hydrated, particularly while taking vitamins in powdered form.

6. **Monitor Your Progress**

Keep a notebook to chart your supplement consumption and any changes in your health, energy levels, or weight reduction progress. This data may help you make educated modifications to your program.

7. **Be Patient**

Supplements may take time to exhibit visible results. Patience is crucial. Stick to your schedule and allow your body time to adjust and react favorably.

8. **Address Stomach Issues**

Some people may feel stomach pain while taking vitamins. If this happens, try taking supplements with meals, choosing liquid or chewable versions, or researching supplements developed for simple digestion.

9. **Adapt to your Lifestyle**

Make supplement integration smooth with your lifestyle. If you travel regularly, buy in travel-sized containers or pre-packaged dosages. Find ways that work for you.

10. **Seek Support and Accountability**

Share your supplement journey with a friend or family member who can give support and keep you responsible. It's simpler to keep on track when you have someone to share the experience with.

11. Budget Wisely

Supplements might vary in price. Set a budget and research cost-effective choices that correspond with your objectives and requirements. Remember, quality should not be sacrificed for cheap.

12. Educate Yourself

Continuously educate yourself on the supplements you're using. Stay updated on the latest research and advancements in the area of nutritional supplements.

13. Adjust as Needed

Over time, your requirements may alter. Be open to altering your supplement regimen appropriately. Consult with a healthcare physician if you feel modifications are required.

By applying these tactics and keeping proactive in your approach to supplement integration, you will pass frequent roadblocks and get the full advantages of these essential tools in your weight loss journey.

Long-Term Sustainability: Maintaining a Balanced Approach to Supplements

Your weight reduction journey is not a sprint; it's a lifetime marathon. To preserve and even increase your well-being throughout the years, it's vital to approach the integration of supplements with balance and a long-term view.

Think beyond merely dropping pounds and explore the bigger canvas of your entire health. Supplements should be seen as lifetime friends on this trip. Here's how:

Sustainability: Choose supplements that are sustainable for the long run. Focus on those that promote your total health and vitality, not simply speedy weight reduction. Your selections should endure the test of time.

Regular Assessments: Periodically reassess your supplement regimen. As your life develops, so do your health requirements. Consult with healthcare providers to ensure your selections stay suitable.

Comprehensive Health: Shift your emphasis from basic weight reduction to comprehensive health. Supplements are merely one component of the puzzle. Balance is obtained by a mix of nutritious eating, regular exercise, mental well-being, and stress management.

Preventative Approach: Look to supplements as a form of prevention. Many nutrients contribute to long-term well-being and may lessen your risk of chronic illnesses.

Avoiding Overuse: Refrain from overusing supplements. Excessive ingestion might lead to imbalances or significant health hazards. Always stick to suggested doses.

Entire Foods: Remember that entire foods should form the cornerstone of your diet. Supplements are supposed to complement your diet, not replace it. Aim for a broad and nutrient-rich dietary consumption.

Physical Activity: Maintain an active lifestyle. Physical exercise is vital for lifetime health. It not only boosts the efficiency of vitamins but also adds to general well-being.

Mindful Practices: Embrace awareness via meditation, yoga, or stress reduction approaches. These activities assist mental and emotional well-being, supplementing the physical parts of your lifetime journey.

Detoxification: Consider periodic detoxification programs to clear your body of stored poisons. Consult with healthcare specialists to guarantee safe and effective procedures.

Accountability and Assistance: Stay accountable to your health objectives by seeking assistance and establishing friendships with like-minded others. Sharing your journey with others may be motivational.

Personalization: Recognize that your lifetime path is uniquely yours. Customize your strategy based on your specific requirements, interests, and health state.

Continuous Learning: Stay updated about the newest breakthroughs in nutrition and supplements. Knowledge helps you to make educated decisions as you progress on your path.

Enjoy the Process: Lastly, appreciate the ride. Lifelong health is not about perpetual sacrifice but about finding pleasure and satisfaction in your choices. It's about accepting a balanced and sustainable approach to well-being.

Your trip is a lifetime experience, and supplements are tools that may help you navigate it effectively. By keeping balance and a long-term perspective, you'll not only accomplish weight reduction but also encourage permanent well-being.

Real Success Stories: Women Who Thrived with Supplements

Meet Sarah: A Journey of Renewed Energy

Sarah, a busy professional and mother of two, found it challenging to get rid of those post-pregnancy pounds. Despite her best attempts, her energy levels were at an all-time low. Feeling disappointed, she sought help and found the power of vitamins.

"After I began taking vitamins that matched my requirements, it felt like a cloud had lifted. I had more energy to run after my kids and be productive at work. The increase in my metabolism from specific vitamins made a considerable impact on my weight reduction quest. It wasn't a miracle remedy, but it provided the additional support I needed to finally see progress. And most significantly, I felt like myself again."

Jane's Journey to a Balanced Life

Jane, a fitness fanatic, discovered that her strenuous exercises were taking a toll on her body. She went to vitamins to assist her health and recuperation.

"I was pushing my body hard in the gym, but I realized I needed to consider my entire wellness. Supplements like protein and BCAAs were my training buddies. They helped me grow and restore muscle, minimizing discomfort and tiredness. I could feel the change in my exercises, and it was empowering. Integrating these supplements into my regimen helped me to find a balance between pushing my boundaries and taking care of my body."

These testimonies are just two instances of the innumerable women who have successfully incorporated supplements into their routines, accomplishing their health and weight reduction objectives. Their tales highlight the transforming power of individualized supplement regimens when paired with a dedication to holistic well-being.

Your Unique Journey: Customizing Your Approach

In the realm of weight reduction, no two roads are alike. Your path is uniquely yours, molded by your objectives, interests, and particular requirements. Embracing your distinctiveness and adapting your approach is a crucial element to success.

Whether your target is dramatic weight reduction, a better lifestyle, or minor changes, your method should correspond with your unique aims. Your food choices should reflect your likes and preferences. If you have dietary limitations or practice a certain eating style, consider supplements and recipes that accord with your culinary preferences.

Exercise should be a source of delight, not fear. Select physical activities that appeal to you, whether it's dancing, trekking, or practicing yoga. When you love your exercise, you're more likely to remain dedicated and consistent.

Supplement choices should be guided by your particular demands. Consult a healthcare practitioner to discover any vitamin deficits or particular health issues. Tailor your supplement options to meet these particular challenges.

Mindfulness activities and stress reduction approaches should connect with your personality. Experiment with various approaches to find what fits you best, whether it's conventional meditation, mindful coloring, journaling, or just spending peaceful minutes in nature.

The technique you use to monitor your success should coincide with your unique style. Some folks thrive on extensive monitoring tools, while others prefer the simplicity of a notebook. Personalize your tracking method to make it a relevant part of your trip.

Whether you find strength in social support or prefer a self-guided approach, your support system should match your social style. Adapt to problems as they emerge, because they are part of every trip.

Celebrate your individuality throughout your journey. Your journey is unlike anybody else's, and that distinctiveness is what makes your successes genuinely valuable. By personalizing your strategy, you not only attain your weight reduction objectives but also start on a meaningful and sustainable trip that's entirely your own.

Remember, your trip is your artwork; personalize it, accept it, and relish every second of it.

CHAPTER 4

Dispelling Common Misconceptions about Natural Supplements

As you commence on your road of integrating natural supplements into your weight loss strategy, it's crucial to be aware of and debunk some common myths that typically surround these products. Here are a few myths:

1. **Myth**: Natural Means Safe
- **Reality**: While many natural supplements are safe when used carefully, not all of them are devoid of potential side effects or interactions with pharmaceuticals. Always contact a healthcare practitioner before introducing new supplements, especially if you have underlying health concerns or are using drugs.

2. **Myth**: Supplements Guarantee Rapid Results
- **Reality**: Natural supplements can complement your weight reduction efforts, but they are not

miracle pills that guarantee fast results. Sustainable weight reduction involves a mix of elements, including a balanced diet, frequent exercise, and patience.

3. **Myth**: More Is Better
- **Reality**: Excessive use of supplements can lead to imbalances and severe consequences. Always follow suggested amounts, and avoid overloading your system with various substances without expert assistance.

4. **Myth**: Supplements Replace a Healthy Diet
- **Reality**: Supplements should never replace a balanced diet. They are supposed to augment, not supersede, your dietary choices. Whole foods supply a wide diversity of nutrients and should form the foundation of your diet.

5. **Myth**: Supplements Are a One-Size-Fits-All Solution
- **Reality**: Everyone's dietary demands are distinct. What works for one individual may not work for another. Personalization is crucial when

picking supplements to suit specific needs and health objectives.

6. **Myth**: Supplements Can Compensate for Poor Lifestyle Habits
- **Reality**: Supplements cannot substitute for an unhealthy lifestyle. They function most well when integrated into a comprehensive program that includes a balanced diet, exercise, stress management, and proper sleep.

7. **Myth**: Supplements Are Unregulated
- **Reality**: In many countries, dietary supplements are subject to regulation to guarantee safety and quality. Look for items that hold certificates from trustworthy organizations, and always purchase from trusted suppliers.

8. **Myth**: All Natural Supplements Are Equally Effective
- **Reality**: The efficacy of natural supplements might vary greatly. Factors like quality, purity, and formulation play a crucial influence.

Research and pick items based on research and expert recommendations.

9. **Myth**: Supplements Are Only for Weight Loss
- **Reality**: Supplements offer a broad variety of health applications beyond weight reduction. Some assist mental health, some increase physical performance, and many contribute to general wellness.

10. **Myth**: Supplements Alone Are a Comprehensive Solution
- **Reality**: Supplements are one element of the jigsaw. Comprehensive well-being covers variables such as mental health, stress management, and physical activity. A balanced approach is crucial for success.

By debunking these common misunderstandings, you're better able to make informed decisions about integrating natural supplements into your weight reduction journey. Remember that information, paired with a holistic approach to health, is your greatest advantage.

The Evolving Landscape of Natural Supplements: Trends and Insights

Here, we investigate some major trends and ideas impacting the landscape of natural supplements:

1. Personalization

Personalized nutrition is at the forefront of supplement developments. Advances in genetics and data analysis allow for personalized supplement recommendations based on an individual's unique genetic composition and health profile. This tendency underscores the significance of accuracy in supplement selection.

2. Transparency and Quality

Consumers are increasingly seeking transparency and quality assurance from supplement makers. Certifications and third-party testing for purity and potency have become necessary. Brands that achieve these requirements are earning trust and loyalty.

3. Natural Components

The trend for natural and plant-based components continues to rise. Consumers prefer supplements manufactured from real foods and plants, free from artificial ingredients, colors, and fillers.

4. Sustainability

Environmental concern is impacting supplement selections. Sustainable sourcing of ingredients, eco-friendly packaging, and ethical procedures in the supplement sector are becoming more crucial issues for customers.

5. Gut Health

The relationship between gut health and general well-being is increasing awareness. Probiotics, prebiotics, and supplements that assist digestive health are on the rise as consumers attempt to optimize their microbiomes.

6. Immune Support

Recent global events have raised interest in supplements that support immune function. Vitamins like C and D, as well as minerals like zinc, have gained increased appeal due to their possible immune-boosting qualities.

7. Mental Wellness

Mental health supplements, especially those targeting stress reduction, mood improvement, and cognitive support, are witnessing heightened demand as consumers pursue holistic well-being.

8. Aging Gracefully

Anti-aging vitamins are a developing area as individuals attempt to retain energy and health as they age. Collagen supplements, antioxidants, and minerals that assist joint and bone health are in the limelight.

9. CBD and Hemp-Based Products

Cannabidiol (CBD) and hemp-based supplements continue to garner attention for their potential therapeutic advantages, notably in controlling pain, anxiety, and sleep difficulties.

10. Sustainable Weight Management

Weight management supplements that match with sustainable, long-term approaches to health are predicted to stay important. Consumers are seeking solutions that help progressive, sustained weight loss and general well-being.

11. Digital Health Integration

Technology is playing a role in supplement recommendations and tracking. Apps and gadgets that monitor health parameters and give individualized supplement advice are being developed.

12. Regulatory Changes

Regulatory bodies are regularly changing recommendations for dietary supplements. Staying updated about these changes is vital for both consumers and producers to guarantee product safety and efficacy.

As the landscape of natural supplements continues to expand, consumers must stay informed, seek expert help, and make decisions matched with their personal health goals. The path of incorporating supplements into your weight reduction strategy is part of this dynamic and fascinating environment, bringing new opportunities for better well-being.

Key Takeaways
- Holistic well-being is the ultimate objective of your weight reduction quest.
- Natural supplements are great aids when combined properly.
- Personalization, openness, and quality are key in supplement selection.
- Sustainable decisions and gradual growth lead to enduring well-being.

Conclusion
Embrace Your Lifelong Journey to Well-Being

Your quest for weight loss and well-being is a lifelong endeavor. Every day gives us a chance to make decisions that lead to enduring health and energy. Remember, it's not just about numbers on a scale; it's about nourishing your health, embracing balance, and discovering the greatest version of yourself.

As you conclude this book, keep with you the awareness that you have the tools, the insight, and the strength to go on your road to well-being. Natural supplements are your allies, but your devotion to balanced eating, regular physical exercise, mental well-being, and individuality will be your guiding light.

Embrace the trip with confidence, and may each day be a reminder that you have the capacity to build your own route to wellness. You've got this!